CONTENTS

Surveys in Great Britain[1] indicate that swimming is a very popular activity with recreational groups. The Amateur Swimming Association and the Royal Life Saving Society, through their award schemes, have tried to encourage active participation. The aim of this programme is not only to encourage people to embark on a regular training programme (i.e. 3 or 4 times a week) but to help them to understand how to construct their own workouts. Training terms are explained, a focus is given and many kinds of training aid are used.

Training results in an increased capacity of both cardiac and skeletal muscle to utilise oxygen for energy production. The greater the aerobic capacity of skeletal muscle the more the onset of fatigue is delayed. There is a metabolic shift from the use of carbohydrates as the main fuel towards a greater utilisation of fats; it is the use of carbohydrates in providing the fuel for energy production in muscle that is associated with fatiguing by-products (i.e. lactic acid). In the present context health, or fitness, is defined as the ability to endure, as this reflects an efficient cardiovascular and metabolic system.

INTENSITY

Training means working at an intensity greater than that achieved during a normal working day. In swimming a person can exercise and improve the aerobic system by either (i) swims lasting longer than 3 minutes at a moderate pace; or (ii) repeated swims at various distances (interval type training) where the intensity of the swim is approximately 75–80% of maximum speed for a particular distance and the rest intervals are as half as long as the time taken to swim the distance.[2]

If a person increases the intensity of the swims to

[1] Duffield, B.S. *et al.* (1983) *A Digest of Sports Statistics*, 1st edn. London: Sports Council.
[2] Troup, J. and Reese, R. (1983) *A Scientific Approach to the Sport of Swimming*. Gainesville: Scientific Sports.

HEALTH EDUCATION AUTHORITY

Inverclyde Libraries

34106 001789143

Acknowledgements   The author acknowledges the assistance of Professor C. Williams and the use of his research facilities at the Department of Physical Education and Sports Science, Loughborough University of Technology.

Photographs by Roddy Paine

British Library Cataloguing in Publication Data
Hardy, Colin A.
  Swimming for fitness.
  1. Physical fitness. Swimming
  I. Title
  613.7′1

  ISBN 0 340 52510 X

First published 1990

Typeset by Wearside Tradespools, Fulwell, Sunderland
Printed in Great Britain for the educational publishing division of Hodder and Stoughton Ltd, Mill Road, Dunton Green, Sevenoaks, Kent by Thomson Litho Ltd, East Kilbride

above 90% of maximum speed,[3] increased muscle lactic acid levels impair the function of the muscle and, ultimately, swimming speed. Although such anaerobic exercise is unnecessary for fitness programmes, some faster efforts have been included in the present programme to give people practical experience of this energy system.

The suggested target heart rate for training the aerobic system can vary between 120 and 170 beats per minute.[3] The American Heart Association recommend target zones of 60–75% of maximum heart rate, increasing, if the person so wishes, to 85% after 6 months or more of regular exercise (Table 1).[4] The easiest place to check the pulse rate is the carotid artery in the neck; count the number of beats for 6 seconds and add a zero.

Table 1   Recommended target heart rates and mean maximum heart rates in a swimming programme

Age (years)	Target zone (beats per min) (60–75%)	Mean maximum (100%)
20	120–150	200
25	117–146	195
30	114–142	190
35	111–138	185
40	108–135	180
45	105–131	175
50	102–127	170
55	99–123	165
60	96–120	160
65	93–116	155
70	90–113	150

Reproduced from reference 4 with permission of The American Heart Association

MOBILITY

Gentle stretching movements to the end-position (i.e. point of tightness) can loosen up the joints before starting a swimming workout. Over a period of time the combined effect of stretching exercises and performing the various kicking and pulling actions can improve or maintain the range of movement in a joint.

[3] Maglischo, E.W. and Brennan, C. (1985) *Swim for the Health of It*. London: Mayfield Publishing.
[4] American Heart Association (1984) *Swimming for a Healthy Heart*. Dallas: American Heart Association's Office of Communications.

PARTICIPANT OBJECTIVES

1. Improve fitness through the medium of swimming.
2. Understand the contribution of swimming training methods to fitness.
3. Develop the ability to work with others in preparing a swimming programme.
4. Develop the ability to prepare a personal swimming programme.

THE PROGRAMME FOR HEALTH

In general, a swimming programme tends to follow a distinct developmental pattern. Firstly, there is the step of learning to swim – the participant masters the stages of familiarisation, orientation and controlled propulsion. Secondly, there is the step of developing swimming ability in various situations – experiencing and improving the watermanship skills. Finally, there is the commitment to swimming that depends upon the effectiveness of steps one and two, available opportunities and the dominant social pressures. The swimming programme presented here is part of the watermanship experiences. It is to be hoped any eventual commitment to swimming will include such a fitness element (Fig. 1).

WHO SHOULD PARTICIPATE?

The programme is for anyone who is of the appropriate swimming level. It will probably start with people aged 14 years and over who are ready for watermanship experiences.

LEVELS I TO IV

People can enter the programme at either Levels I or II depending upon previous swimming experience and general fitness. However, progress to Levels III and IV must be based on experience of the previous level. A swimmer who varies considerably in the performance of the strokes may be working at two levels depending upon the emphasis of the workout.

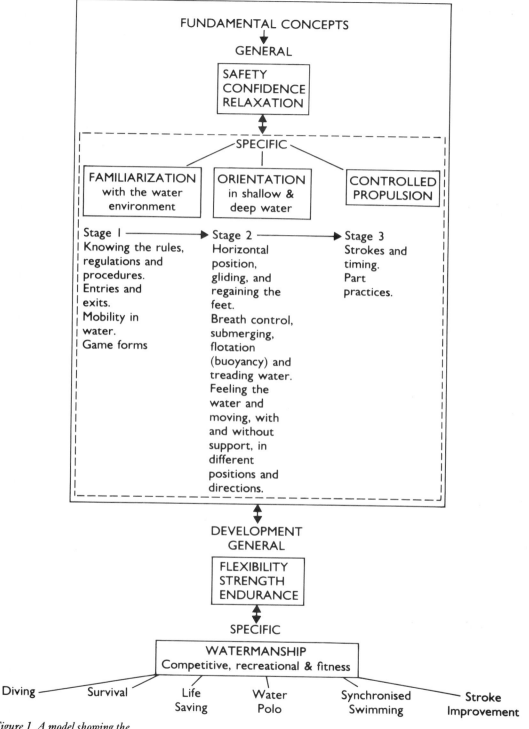

FUNDAMENTAL CONCEPTS
↓
GENERAL

SAFETY
CONFIDENCE
RELAXATION
↕
SPECIFIC

FAMILIARIZATION
with the water
environment

ORIENTATION
in shallow &
deep water

CONTROLLED
PROPULSION

Stage 1 ⟶
Knowing the rules,
regulations and
procedures.
Entries and
exits.
Mobility in
water.
Game forms

Stage 2 ⟶
Horizontal
position,
gliding, and
regaining the
feet.
Breath control,
submerging,
flotation
(buoyancy) and
treading water.
Feeling the
water and
moving, with
and without
support, in
different
positions and
directions.

Stage 3
Strokes and
timing.
Part
practices.

↕
DEVELOPMENT
GENERAL

FLEXIBILITY
STRENGTH
ENDURANCE
↕
SPECIFIC

WATERMANSHIP
Competitive, recreational & fitness

Diving — Survival   Life
Saving   Water
Polo   Synchronised
Swimming — Stroke
Improvement

*Figure 1 A model showing the
development of swimming.
(Reproduced from Swim (1987),*
Spring, *4–7, by permission of The
Institute of Swimming Teachers and
Coaches.)*

SAFETY

It is essential:

1. To have some understanding of life-saving procedures and the ability to act in an emergency and perform expired air resuscitation.

2. To swim in properly supervised pools and to adhere to the swimming pool regulations (e.g. dive in the deep end only) and routines (e.g. shower before entering the water).

GETTING STARTED

1. Active teenagers and adults with some swimming experience may enter at either Level I or Level II.

2. Inactive teenagers and adults with some swimming experience should enter at Level I, and only after passing a medical examination by their local medical practitioner.

3. If during the testing (see instructions for Levels I and II) a person experiences any unusual sensations (e.g. a sharp pain in the neck, chest, shoulder or arm; or feelings of lightheadedness or dizziness) the test must be stopped and the local medical practitioner seen before continuing with the swimming programme.

PERFORMANCE ORGANISATION

1. Place the swimmers in lanes according to their level and group.

2. Give each person a workout according to the distance achieved.

3. To avoid collisions organise adjacent lanes to swim in opposing directions.

4. Place appropriate equipment at the end of each lane.

5. Ensure that all participants can see a pace clock (or a watch with a second hand).

6. As people progress encourage them to select their own workout from the swimming programme.

7. Once people understand the demands of the swimming programme they should be encouraged to prepare their own workouts in groups or as individuals.

HOW TO PRESENT THE WORKOUTS

Once the workout has been decided upon, it must be presented in an abbreviated form that can be read and understood easily. For groups, the workout details could either be placed on a black or white board or displayed on a wall using an overhead projector. Individual workout details can be written in *biro* on a card, wrapped in a plastic covering and then placed flat on the pool side. Alternatively, the details can be written on a sheet of paper, which when dipped in water, will stick to the edge of the pool (see Appendix A).

HOW TO ADAPT THE PROGRAMME

If swimming conditions and timetabling do not permit the development of the complete programme, best use of the resources may be achieved by the following:

1. (a) Try out selected aspects with one or more groups working across the width of the pool
   (b) If times are needed for interval-type practices, the time will have to be based on the performance of an average member of the group.

2. Use the programme as a guide and resource pack for other parts of the swimming curriculum (e.g. the focus and question section in each workout can be used for stroke improvement).

At all times be prepared to adapt the material and to encourage and help groups who wish to start their own programme.

GOGGLES

Swimming goggles should be used to improve participants' vision and to reduce eye irritations. It may take several workouts to get the goggles properly adjusted but it is important to persevere. Special anti-fog goggles can be purchased. In all cases the schools must adhere to any local education authority rules on this matter.

TRAINING AIDS

Although training aids are not essential for the completion of a workout, they do give variety to the swimming programme (Fig. 2).

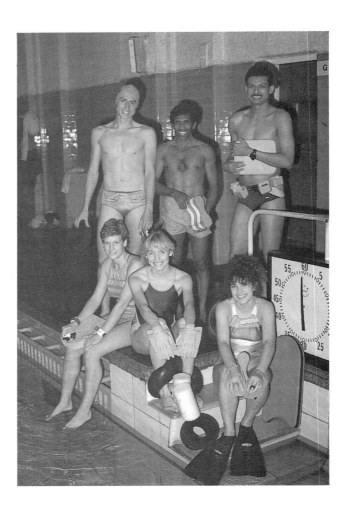

Figure 2 The training aids shown are: kick board, pull buoy, hand paddles, wrist weights, training tube, drag suit, drag belt, drag ring, fins, small pace clock.

THE SWIMMING STROKES

The strokes used in the programme are:

- Breast stroke.
- Back crawl.
- Front crawl.
- Side stroke.
- Butterfly dolphin.
- Elementary back stroke.
- Butterfly breast stroke.
- 'Old English' back stroke.
- Inverted breast stroke.
- Trudgeon stroke.
- Breast stroke in the supine position.

Although the four competitive strokes of the breast stroke, back crawl, front crawl and butterfly dolphin form the basis of the programme, the other strokes will help to maintain interest in the work. Fuller details of the strokes can be found in other swimming texts.[5-7]

[5] Hardy, C.A. (1987) *Handbook for the Teacher of Swimming*. London: Pelham Books.
[6] Department of Education (1981) *Swimming*. Wellington, New Zealand: Department of Education.
[7] Vickers, B.J. and Vincent, W.J. (1984) *Swimming*, 4th edn. Dubuque: Wm. C. Brown Co.

Breast stroke

The arm and legs are both moved in a simultaneous and symmetrical pattern. From an extended position in front of the head the arms are moved downwards, backwards and outwards to a position just in front of the shoulder line. (The stronger swimmers will bend at the elbow during the pull.) As the hands are circled inwards and upwards towards the chin, the feet are brought upwards to the seat and the knees are moved forwards and outwards. The arms are then stretched forwards beneath the water surface and, with the feet turned outwards, a vigorous circular kick is made. The next stroke may begin immediately or a short glide may be held in the stretched position.

A breath can be taken to the front during the arm pull (weaker swimmers) or at the end of the pull (stronger swimmers). Breathing out occurs during the arm recovery stage.

Figure 3

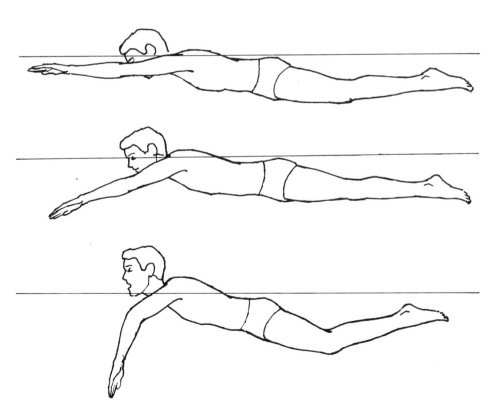

Pull and breathe

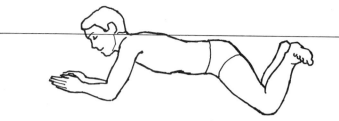

Recover the arms and the legs

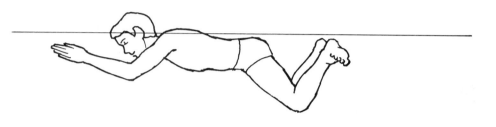

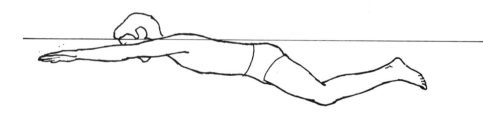

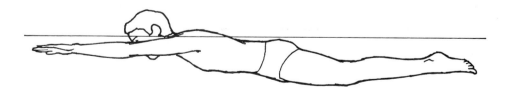

Kick and stretch the arms

Focus   PULL – RECOVER ARMS AND LEGS – KICK
AND STRETCH ARMS

Back crawl

The arms are moved in a continuous windmill-type action with a straight and high arm recovery and a straight or bent arm ('S') pull. The arm is placed into the water in an extended position beyond the head, close to the centre line with the palm facing outwards. The pull ends with the arms straight and close to the side.

The leg kick is an alternating up and down movement just below the water surface. The kick is initiated from the hips and there is some knee bend at the end of the downbeat.

Breathing is not a problem in back crawl but breathing in as one arm recovers and breathing out as the other arm recovers is a common rhythm.

The swimmer usually kicks six times to every arm cycle.

Figure 4

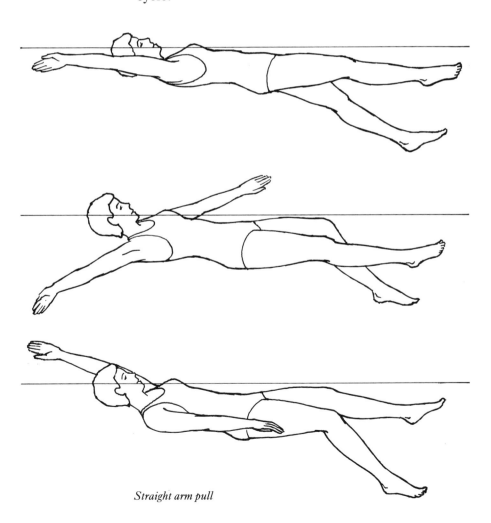

Straight arm pull

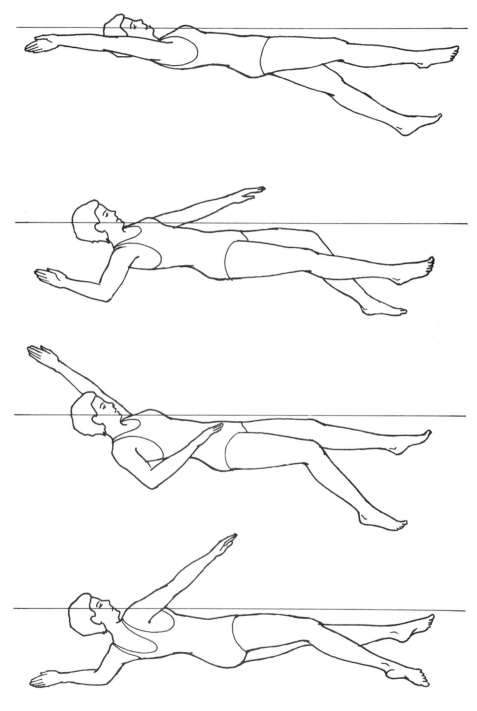

'S' pull

Focus   STEADY BUT CONTINUOUS ARM AND LEG
ACTIONS

Front crawl

The arms are moved in a continuous and alternating action. The slightly bent arm is placed into the water beyond the head and close to the centre line with the fingertips leading. The hand is then pulled backwards in a curved path to the thigh and recovered in a controlled upwards and forwards action. The arm is increasingly bent during the first part of the recovery and gradually straightened for the almost extended entry.

The leg kick is an alternating up and down movement just below the water surface. The kick is initiated from the hips and there is some knee bend at the end of the upbeat.

A breath is taken to the side when one arm is forwards and the other is backwards, and it is to the side of the arm that is backwards. Breathing out occurs when the face is downwards.

The swimmer usually kicks six times to each arm cycle but there are several variations including two-beat and cross-over kicks.

Figure 5

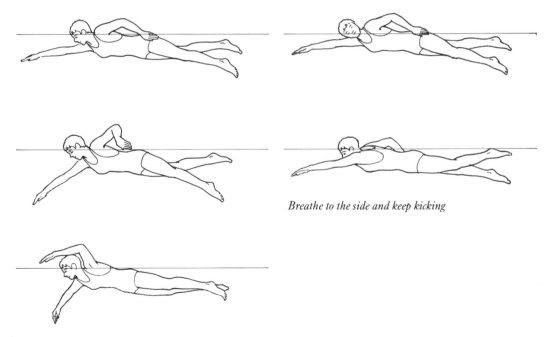

Breathe to the side and keep kicking

Recover the arms with a high elbow

Focus   STEADY BUT CONTINUOUS ARM, LEG AND
BREATHING ACTIONS

Side stroke

As the top hand is recovered beneath the water surface from the thigh to below the chin, the bottom hand is pulled from the extended position in front of the head to a position just below the top hand. During the coming together of the hands, the legs are bent and spread in a sideways direction. The push back of the top hand and the stretch forwards of the bottom hand coincide with the straightening and coming together of the legs. Usually a short glide is held in this side-lying and streamlined position.

A breath is taken to the side as the bottom arm pulls. Breathing out occurs as the bottom arm is stretched forwards.

Figure 6

Pull with the left arm and recover the right arm and the legs

Push with the right arm and kick with the legs

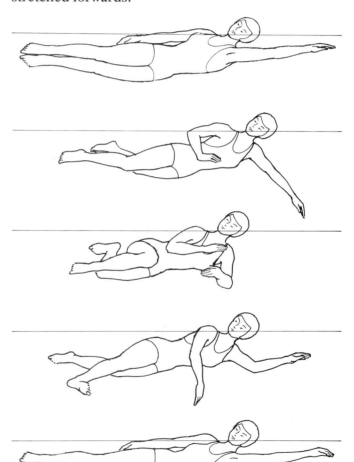

Focus

RECOVER LEGS AND BRING HANDS TOGETHER – KICK LEGS AND PART HANDS

Butterfly dolphin

The arms are moved over and through the water in a simultaneous and symmetrical pattern. The slightly bent arms are placed into the water beyond the head, near the shoulder lines and with the fingertips leading. The hands are then pulled backwards in a curved path to the thighs and recovered in a low circular swing over the water surface.

The up and down kick is initiated from the hips, and there is some knee bend at the end of the upbeat.

A breath can be taken to the front during the arm pull (weaker swimmers) or at the end of the pull (stronger swimmers). Breathing out occurs when the face is downwards.

The swimmer usually kicks twice to each arm cycle; the first downbeat comes as the arms start to pull and the second downbeat coincides with the last part of the pull. Sometimes, with the weaker swimmer, there is a delay in starting the next arm pull because more time is needed to complete the second leg beat.

Figure 7

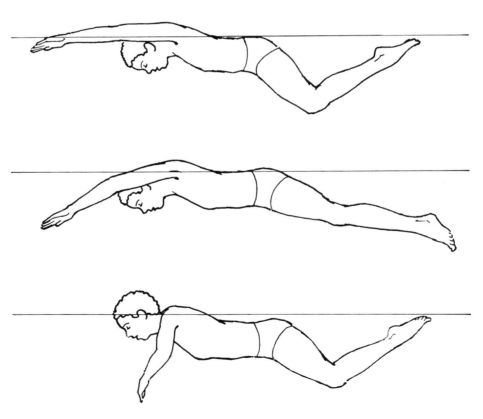

Pull and kick

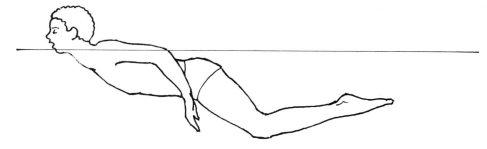

Push back and breathe

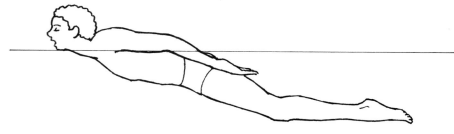

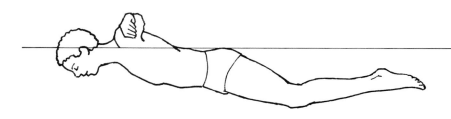

Recover the arms and drop the head

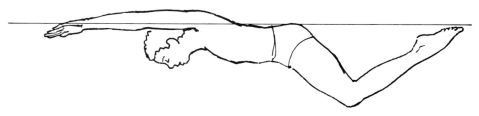

Focus   DEFINITE LEG BEAT WITH A LONG ARM
PULL

Elementary back stroke

The arms and legs are both moved in a simultaneous and symmetrical pattern. From an extended 'Y' position the arms are pulled sideways to the thighs, then recovered bent along the body to the shoulders and stretched back to the starting position. The arms remain below the water surface throughout the arm cycle. As the arms are recovered and stretched the heels are brought towards the seat and the knees taken upwards and outwards. The feet are then turned outwards and the arm pull coincides with a vigorous circular leg kick. The kick is usually completed before the pull, and a glide is held with the legs together, feet together and the arms by the sides.

A breath is taken during the recovery of the arms and legs. Breathing out occurs during the kick and pull.

Figure 8

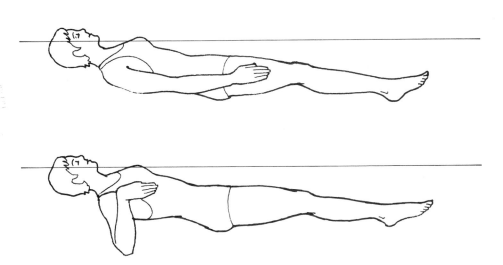

Recover the arms close to the body

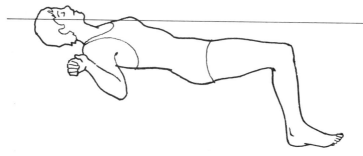

Recover the legs and move the arms to a 'Y' position

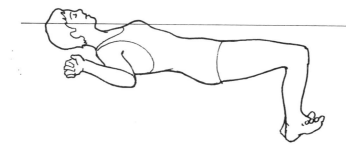

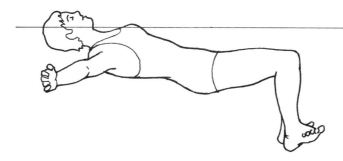

Kick and pull

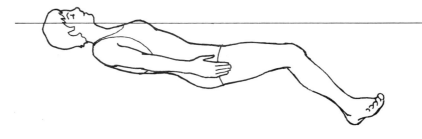

Focus   **RECOVER ARMS AND LEGS – KICK AND
PULL**

Butterfly breast stroke

The arms are moved over and through the water in a simultaneous and symmetrical pattern. The slightly bent arms are placed into the water beyond the head, near the shoulder lines and with the fingertips leading. The hands are then pulled backwards in a curved path to the thighs and recovered in a low circular swing over the water surface. During the first part of the arm recovery the feet are brought upwards to the seat and the knees are moved forwards and outwards. As the arms complete the recovery the feet are turned out and a vigorous circular leg kick is made. The next stroke may begin immediately or a short glide may be held in the stretched position using a slightly different timing.

A breath is taken to the front during the early part of the arm pull. Breathing out occurs when the face is downwards.

Figure 9

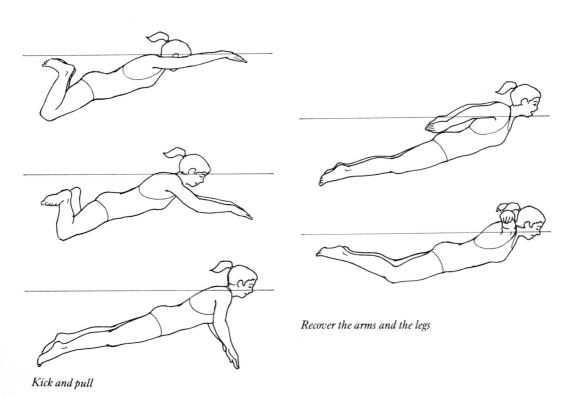

Recover the arms and the legs

Kick and pull

Focus   RECOVER ARMS AND LEGS – KICK AND PULL

'Old English' back
stroke

The arms and legs are both moved in a simultaneous and symmetrical pattern. From an extended position together and beyond the head the arms are pulled sideways to the thighs. As the arms are recovered straight and high over the water surface the heels are brought towards the seat and the knees taken upwards and outwards. When the arms are about to pull, the circular kicking action with the feet turned outwards will have already started. A glide is usually held with the legs together, feet extended and the arms by the sides.

A breath is taken during the recovery of the arms and legs. Breathing out occurs during the kick and pull.

Figure 10

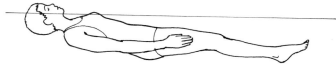

Lift the arms upwards

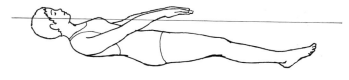

Enter the arms beyond the head, kick and pull

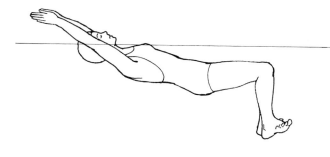

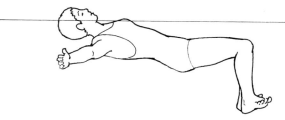

Focus   **RECOVER ARMS AND LEGS – KICK AND PULL**

Inverted breast stroke

The arms and legs are both moved in a simultaneous and symmetrical pattern. From an extended position together and beyond the head the arms are pulled sideways to the thighs. As the bent arms are recovered along the body to the shoulders and beneath the water surface, the heels are brought towards the seat and the knees taken upwards and outwards. The arms are then stretched forwards beyond the head and, with the feet turned outwards, a vigorous circular kick is made. The next stroke may begin immediately or a short glide may be held in the stretched position.

A breath is taken during the first part of the arm recovery. Breathing out occurs during the stretch forwards of the arm beyond the head.

Figure 11

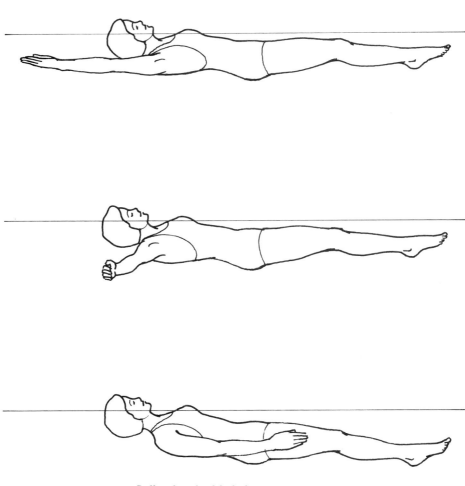

Pull to the side of the body

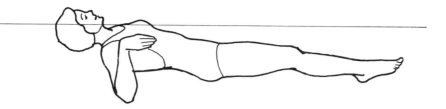

Recover the arms close to the body, and recover the legs

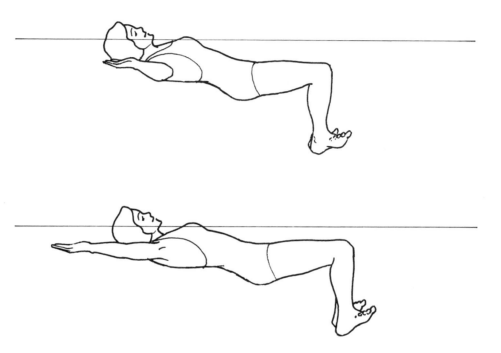

Kick and stretch the arms beyond the head

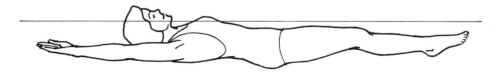

Focus   **PULL – RECOVER LEGS AND MOVE HANDS TO SHOULDERS – KICK AND STRETCH ARMS**

Trudgeon stroke

This is a combination of a front crawl arm action with either a breast stroke or side stroke leg movement. It is usual to recover and kick the legs once to every arm cycle, although it is possible to recover and kick twice with the legs.

A breath is taken to the side when one arm is forwards and the other is backwards, and it is to the side of the arm that is backwards. Breathing out occurs when the face is downwards.

This is a stroke that you can experiment with, and you will probably develop your own timing rhythm.

Figure 12

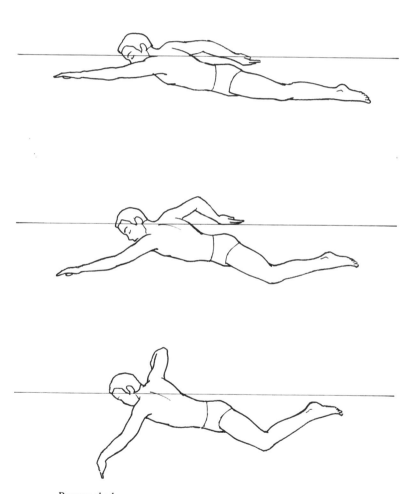

Recover the legs

Kick and breathe to the side

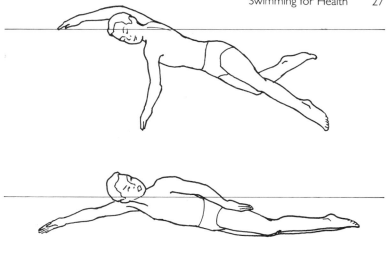

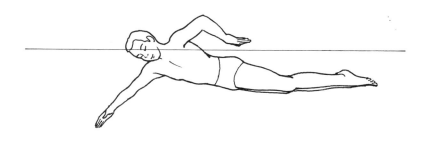

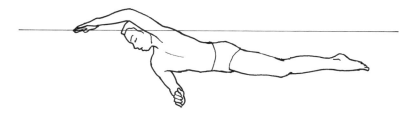

Wait and prepare for the next leg recovery

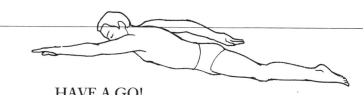

HAVE A GO!

Breast stroke kick in the supine (back) position

The legs are moved continuously in a simultaneous and symmetrical pattern. The heels are brought towards the seat and the knees taken upwards and outwards. With the feet turned outwards, a vigorous circular leg kick is made. A continuous sculling movement with the hands can help the swimmer's propulsion.

A breath is taken regularly at will.

Figure 13

Recover the legs

Turn the feet outwards and kick

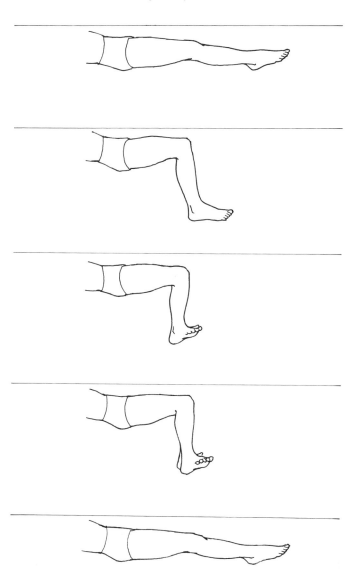

Focus   VIGOROUS CIRCULAR KICK

LEVEL I (100 METRES TO 500 METRES)

If you can swim safely in deep water, let's get started.

INSTRUCTIONS

1. Select your best stroke from back crawl, front crawl and breast stroke.

2. See how far you can swim on your selected stroke without stopping and without getting exhausted (maximum 500 metres).

3. Use the distance achieved as your workout distance.

4. Check for distance improvement after five workouts.

CONTENT

1. *Main stroke*: from back crawl, front crawl and breast stroke.

2. *Other strokes*: side stroke, elementary back stroke and breast stroke kick in the supine position.

3. *Part practices*: kicking and pulling.

4. *Open and spin turns*: on back crawl, front crawl and breast stroke.

5. *Other skills*: regaining the feet, gliding, sculling and treading water.

EXAMPLE WORKOUTS

1. Swimming workouts should take between 10 and 30 minutes.

2. Distance should only be increased after checking for distance improvement (see instructions).

WORKING INSTRUCTIONS

1. **Warm-up** – Prior to starting the swimming workout, do 5–10 minutes of body stretching activities on the pool side and in the water.

2. **Body joints** – Concentrate on stretching and bending the appropriate joints when practising the various stroke techniques and practices.

3. **Pace** – Maintain a moderate pace; swim the shorter distances faster than the longer ones.

4. **Rest** – Rest for up to 2 minutes between workout phases; you can cut down the rest once you have started swimming regularly.

5. **Repetitions** – The stated number of repetitions is only a guide.

6. **Cool-down** – After the swimming workout swim or walk slowly in the water and then do some body stretching on the pool side to reduce the heart rate and to avoid stiffness.

LEVEL 1 – EXAMPLES

EXAMPLE 1

STROKE: Front crawl.
DISTANCE: 100 metres.
OTHER SKILLS: Sculling.
EQUIPMENT: Float or pull buoy, clock or watch.

Phase	Practice	Focus
1. Walking	Shallow end: walk across the pool practising FRONT CRAWL arms and breathing (1–2 minutes)	Lift the arms over the water surface by bending at the elbows
2. Kicking	Shallow end: hold the pool side and practise FRONT CRAWL kicking (3 sets of 15 seconds)	Initiate the leg movements from the hips
3. Full stroke	Swim 2 × 25 metres on FRONT CRAWL (rest after the first 25 metres)	Work hard from the hips in both the upwards and downwards movements.
4. Sculling	Shallow end: place a float between the upper legs and practise sculling in a supine position (1–2 minutes)	Move the palms inwards and outwards in a vigorous action close to the hips

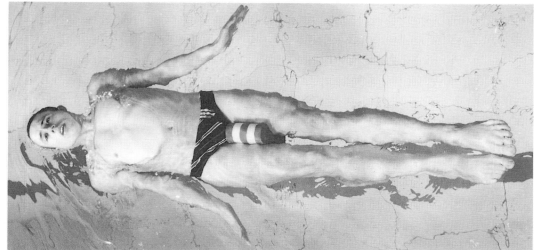

Sculling practice with legs supported by a pull buoy.

5. Full stroke	Swim 2 × 25 metres FRONT CRAWL (rest after the first 25 metres)	Keep the elbows high during the first part of the recovery

QUESTIONS

1. How high did you get the elbows?
2. Did you kick upwards from the hips?
3. Did you keep the legs moving continuously?

4. Did you move head first and feet first?
5. Did you feel the shoulders stretching?

EXAMPLE 2

STROKE: Breast stroke.
DISTANCE: 100 metres.
OTHER SKILLS: Gliding, regaining the feet from the prone position, treading water.
EQUIPMENT: Float or pull buoy.

Phase	Practice	Focus
1. Gliding	Shallow end: push and glide towards the pool side (5 repetitions)	Streamline the body by stretching from the fingertips to the toes
2. Full stroke	Swim 2 × 25 metres on BREAST STROKE (rest after the first 25 metres)	Prepare for an effective kick by bending at the knees and bringing the heels close to the seat
3. Regaining the feet from the prone position	Shallow end: push away from the pool side in the prone position, glide and then stand up (5 repetitions)	Pull down with the arms and bend the legs
4. Treading water	Water at shoulder level: holding a float, tread water (1–2 minutes)	Move the legs in a circular action
5. Full stroke	Swim 2 × 25 metres BREAST STROKE (rest after the first 25 metres)	Stretch and keep the arms beneath the water surface during the arm glide

QUESTIONS

1. Did you feel the tension in the joints?
2. Did you touch the seat with the heels?
3. How quickly did you get to the feet?
4. Did you circle the legs slowly?
5. Did you straighten the arms?

EXAMPLE 3

MAIN STROKE: Front crawl.
SECOND STROKE: Breast stroke.
DISTANCE: 200 metres.
OTHER SKILLS: Gliding and regaining the feet from the prone position, front crawl turn.
EQUIPMENT: Clock or watch.

Phase	Practice	Focus
1. Gliding and regaining the feet from the prone position	Shallow end: push away from the pool side in the prone position, glide and then stand up (5 repetitions)	Stretch and tense the body and limbs

Phase	Practice	Focus
2. Full stroke	Swim 2 × 25 metres on FRONT CRAWL (rest for 20 seconds after the first 25 metres)	Keep the toes pointing backwards
3. Full stroke	Swim 2 × 25 metres on BREAST STROKE (rest for 20 seconds after the first 25 metres)	Kick with the feet turned outwards
4. Turning	Shallow end: swim FRONT CRAWL to the pool side from a distance of 5 metres and practise a spin turn with head up or head down (5 repetitions)	Touch by placing the palm flat against the wall and spin in a tucked position

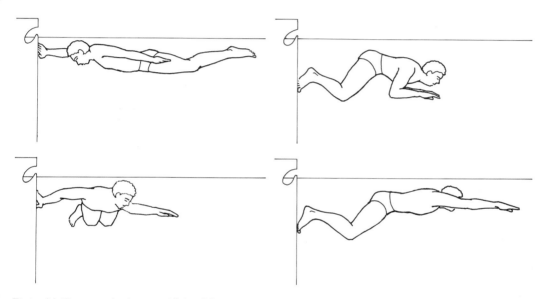

Figure 14 Front crawl spin turn with head down.

5. Full stroke	Swim 2 × 50 metres on FRONT CRAWL (rest for 35 seconds after the 50 metres)	Place the palm flat against the wall and point the fingers in the direction of the turn

QUESTIONS

1. Did you streamline the body?
2. Did you feel the water pressure on the insteps and the soles of feet?
3. Did you feel the water pressure on the insides of the feet?
4. Did you turn smoothly?
5. Did you manage a spin turn?

EXAMPLE 4

STROKE: Back crawl.
DISTANCE: 200 metres.
OTHER SKILLS: Gliding and regaining the feet from the supine position, treading water.
EQUIPMENT: Float or kick board, clock or watch.

Phase	Practice	Focus
1. Gliding and regaining the feet from the supine position	Shallow end: push away from the pool side in the supine position, glide (with the hands by the side) and then stand up (5 repetitions)	Push the hands towards the feet and bend the legs
2. Full stroke	Swim 4 × 25 metres on BACK CRAWL (rest for 20 seconds between each 25 metres)	Recover the arms high over the water surface
3. Part practice	Hold the float above the hips: kick 2 × 25 metres on BACK CRAWL (rest for 25 seconds after the first 25 metres)	Work hard from the hips in both the upwards and downwards movements
4. Treading water	Water at shoulder level: tread water (1–2 minutes)	Move the palms inwards and outwards
5. Full stroke	Swim 50 metres on BACK CRAWL	Stay on the back throughout the turn

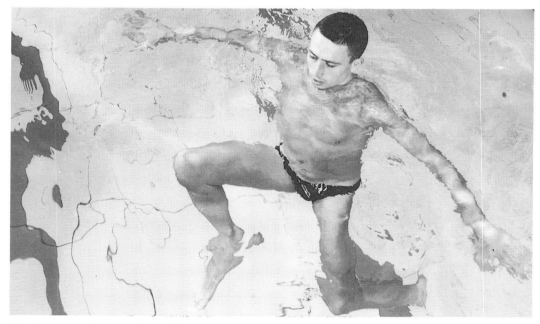

Treading water using an egg-beater kick.

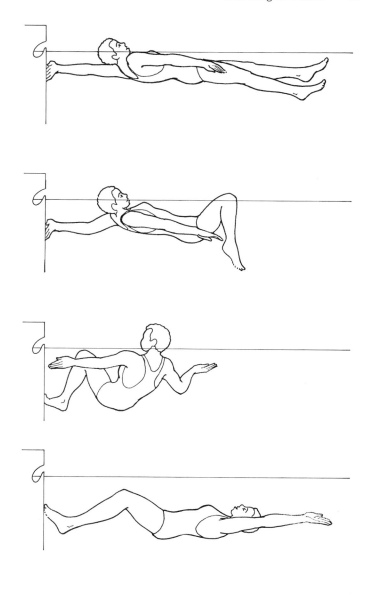

Figure 15 Back crawl spin turn with head out.

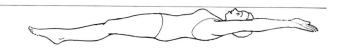

QUESTIONS

1. Did you regain the feet confidently?
2. How close did you get the upper arms to the ears?
3. Did you keep the legs moving continuously and quickly?
4. Did you move the hands slowly?
5. How did you turn at the end of the pool?

EXAMPLE 5

MAIN STROKE: Front crawl.
SECOND STROKE: Back crawl.
DISTANCE: 300 metres.
OTHER SKILLS: Gliding and regaining the feet from the prone position, front crawl turn.
EQUIPMENT: Float or kick board, clock or watch.

Phase	Practice	Focus
1. Gliding and regaining the feet from the prone position	Shallow end: push away from the pool side in the prone position, glide and then stand up (5 repetitions)	Stretch and tense the body and limbs
2. Turning	Shallow end: swim on FRONT CRAWL to the pool side from a distance of 5 metres and practise a spin turn with the head down (5 repetitions)	Spin with the face in the water
3. Full stroke	Swim 100 metres on FRONT CRAWL	Keep the legs and arms moving continuously
4. Full stroke	Swim 4 × 25 metres on BACK CRAWL (rest for 20 seconds between each 25 metres)	Recover the arms high over the water surface
5. Part practice	Hold the float half-way along and extend the arms: kick 2 × 25 metres on FRONT CRAWL (rest for 25 seconds after the first 25 metres)	Concentrate on kicking upwards from the hips
6. Full stroke	Swim 50 metres on FRONT CRAWL	Remember to kick upwards as well as downwards

QUESTIONS

1. How far did you glide?
2. Did you keep the head down?
3. Did you get into a stroke rhythm?
4. Did you enter close to the centre line of the body?
5. Did you keep the feet close to the water surface?
6. Did you keep the legs moving continuously?

EXAMPLE 6

MAIN STROKE: Breast stroke.
SECOND STROKE: Back crawl.
DISTANCE: 300 metres.
OTHER SKILLS: Treading water, breast stroke turn.
EQUIPMENT: Clock or watch.

Phase	Practice	Focus
1. Treading water	Water at shoulder level: tread water (1–2 minutes)	Keep the face just clear of the water and keep the arm and leg movements to a minimum
2. Full stroke	Swim 4 × 25 metres on BREAST STROKE (rest for 20 seconds between each 25 metres)	Sweep the legs round and together in a vigorous movement
3. Full stroke	Swim 4 × 25 metres on BACK CRAWL (rest for 20 seconds between each 25 metres)	Work the legs hard from the hips
4. Turning	Shallow end: swim on BREAST STROKE to the pool side from a distance of 5 metres and practice an open turn (5 repetitions)	Touch the wall with two hands simultaneously, turn, release the hands and sink

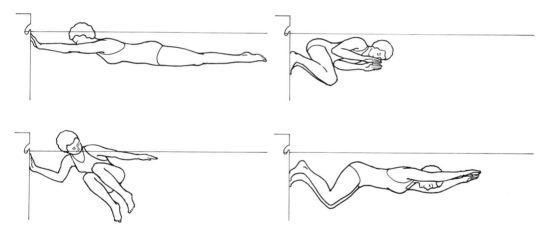

Figure 16 Breast stroke open turn.

5. Full stroke	Swim 100 metres on BREAST STROKE	Turn, release the hands, sink with the hands close to the head and stretch away from the wall

QUESTIONS

1. Did you keep your head back and perform the movements slowly?
2. Did you feel a surge forwards as you kicked?
3. Did your legs ache?
4. Did you release the hands before the feet touched the wall?
5. Did you turn smoothly?

EXAMPLE 7

MAIN STROKE: Back crawl.
SECOND STROKE: Side stroke.
DISTANCE: 400 metres.
OTHER SKILLS: Back crawl turn.
EQUIPMENT: Float or pull buoy, clock or watch.

Phase	Practice	Focus
1. Spinning	Shallow end: practise spinning on the back in a tucked position (5 repetitions of 5 seconds)	Look upwards and spin on the back with the legs in a tucked position
2. Turning	Shallow end: kick, with the turning arm extended beyond the hand, on BACK CRAWL to the pool side from a distance of 5 metres and practise a spin turn (5 repetitions)	Touch with the palm flat against the wall and spin on the back

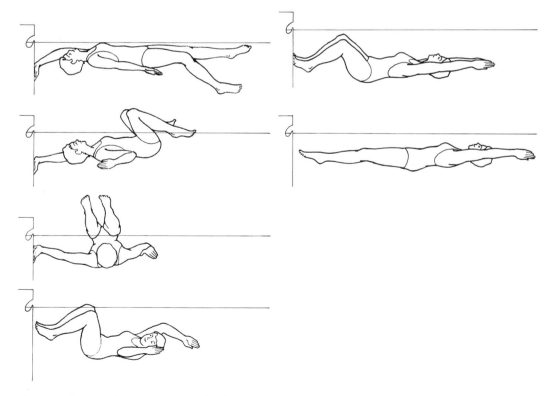

Figure 17 Back crawl spin turn with head under.

Phase	Practice	Focus
3. Full stroke	Swim 200 metres on BACK CRAWL	Keep a steady leg action going with a continuous and controlled arm movement
4. Full stroke	Swim 4 × 25 metres on SIDE STROKE (rest for 20 seconds between each 25 metres)	Look backwards and sideways and keep the body on the side
5. Part practice	Place the float between the upper parts of the legs: pull 2 × 25 metres on BACK CRAWL (rest for 20 seconds after the first 25 metres)	Push, lift and recover the arms in a continuous action
6. Full stroke	Swim 50 metres on BACK CRAWL	Concentrate on keeping the leg action going with a continuous arm movement

QUESTIONS

1. Did you stay on the back?
2. Did you turn smoothly?
3. Did you get into a stroke rhythm?
4. Did you stay on the same side?
5. Did you move from the pull to the recovery continuously?
6. Did you still keep a stroke rhythm?

EXAMPLE 8

MAIN STROKE: Front crawl.
SECOND STROKE: Breast stroke kick in the supine position.
DISTANCE: 400 metres.
OTHER SKILLS: Gliding and regaining the feet from the prone position.
EQUIPMENT: Float or kick board and pull buoy, clock or watch.

Phase	Practice	Focus
1. Gliding and regaining the feet from the prone position	Shallow end: push away from the pool side in the prone position, glide and then stand up (5 repetitions)	Stretch the body and limbs and keep the head down between the arms
2. Kicking	Shallow end: hold the pool side and practise FRONT CRAWL kicking (5 sets of 15 seconds)	Kick from the hips and keep the legs close to the water surface
3. Full stroke	Swim 150 metres on FRONT CRAWL	Lead the pull with the hands and keep the elbows up
4. Full stroke	Swim 4 × 25 metres on BREAST STROKE KICK in the SUPINE POSITION and use a sculling action with the hands	Sweep the legs round and together in a vigorous movement

Phase	Practice	Focus
5. Part position	Place the float between the upper parts of the legs: pull 2 × 25 metres on FRONT CRAWL (rest for 20 seconds after the first 25 metres)	Pull and push back with the hands leading

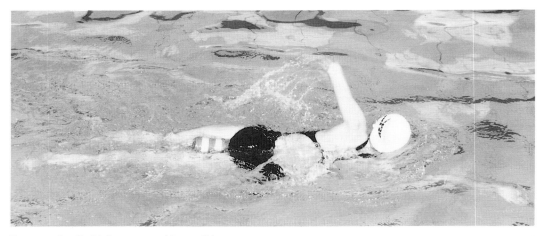

Front crawl pull with legs supported by a pull buoy.

Phase	Practice	Focus
6. Part practice	Hold the float half-way along and extend the arms: kick 2 × 25 metres on FRONT CRAWL (rest for 25 seconds after the first 25 metres)	Keep the legs close to the water surface
7. Full stroke	Swim 50 metres on FRONT CRAWL	Pull and push in a continuous action.

QUESTIONS

1. Did you stretch the joints?
2. Did you keep a fast, shallow action going?
3. Did you feel the pressure on the hands?
4. Did you find it as easy as the breast stroke?
5. Did you feel the pressure on the hands throughout the pull?
6. Did you keep a fast, shallow action going for each 25 metres?
7. How fast did you swim the 50 metres?

EXAMPLE 9

MAIN STROKE: Front crawl, back crawl, breast stroke.
SECOND STROKE: Side stroke, breast stroke kick in the supine position.
DISTANCE: 500 metres.
OTHER SKILLS: Front crawl turn, back crawl turn, breast stroke turn.
EQUIPMENT: Float or kick board, clock or watch.

Phase	Practice	Focus
1. Turning	Shallow end: swim on FRONT CRAWL to the pool side from a distance of 5 metres and practise a spin turn with the head down (5 repetitions)	Touch with the palm flat against the wall and point the fingers in the direction of the turn
2. Full stroke	Swim 100 metres on FRONT CRAWL	Bend and rotate the arms slightly inwards during the pull
3. Turning	Shallow end: kick, with turning arm extended beyond the head, on BACK CRAWL to the pool side from a distance of 5 metres and practise a spin turn (5 repetitions)	Spin on the back, sink with the hands close to the head and stretch away from the wall
4. Full stroke	Swim 100 metres on BACK CRAWL	Keep the wrists firm during the pull and push
5. Turning	Shallow end: swim on BREAST STROKE to the pool side from a distance of 5 metres and practise an open turn (5 repetitions)	Release the hands, sink with the hands close to the head and stretch and glide away from the wall
6. Full stroke	Swim 100 metres on BREAST STROKE	Pull outwards, inwards and forwards in a continuous action
7. Part practice	Hold the float half-way along and extend the arms (prone position) and hold the float above the hips (supine position): kick continuously 4 × 25 metres on 4 strokes (swim 25 metres each on front crawl, back crawl, breast stroke, breast stroke in the supine position in any order)	Keep the feet stretched on front crawl and back crawl and keep the feet hooked and turned outwards on the two breast strokes
8. Full stroke	Swim 100 metres on 4 STROKES; swim 25 metres each on front crawl, back crawl, breast stroke and side stroke in any order	Keep the wrists firm on all strokes during the pull and push

QUESTIONS

1. Did you follow the direction of the fingers?
2. Did you feel the power in the arms?
3. Did you turn confidently on your back?
4. Did you feel the power in the arms?

5. Did you release the hands before the feet touched the wall?
6. Did you 'hold' the water?
7. Did you keep a constant speed going throughout the 25 metres?
8. Did you enjoy the medley swim?

EXAMPLE 10

MAIN STROKE: Breast stroke.
SECOND STROKE: Elementary backstroke, back crawl.
DISTANCE: 500 metres.
OTHER SKILLS: None.
EQUIPMENT: Float or pull buoy, clock or watch.

Phase	Practice	Focus
1. Full stroke	Swim 100 metres on BREAST STROKE	Kick and extend the arms beneath the water surface
2. Full stroke	Swim 100 metres on ELEMENTARY BACK STROKE	Kick as you pull the hands down from a 'Y' position beyond the head
3. Part practice	Place the float between the upper parts of the legs: pull 2 × 25 metres on BREAST STROKE (rest for 20 seconds after the first 25 metres)	Pull outwards and inwards but keep the hands in front of a line dropped from the shoulders
4. Full stroke	Swim 2 × 50 metres on BREAST STROKE (rest for 35 seconds after the first 50 metres)	Pull and recover in a continuous action with the hands remaining in front of a line dropped from the shoulders
5. Full stroke	Swim 100 metres on BACK CRAWL	Keep the feet stretched and just break the water surface with the toes at the end of the upward movement
6. Full stroke	Swim 50 metres on BREAST STROKE	Extend the arms beneath the water surface and pause for a moment

QUESTIONS

1. Did you manage a short glide?
2. Did you get the timing right?
3. Could you see your hands out of the 'corners' of your eyes?

4. Did you feel supported by the arms?
5. Did you manage to break the water surface with the toes?
6. Is a short glide part of your technique?

LEVEL II (600 METRES TO 1000 METRES)

INSTRUCTIONS

1. Select your best two strokes from back crawl, front crawl and breast stroke.

2. On different days, see how far you can swim on your selected strokes without stopping and without getting exhausted (maximum 1000 metres).

3. Use the distance achieved on your strongest stroke as your workout distance.

4. Use the distance achieved on your other stroke as your workout distance for the second main stroke workouts.

5. Check for distance improvement once you feel that a particular workout distance is becoming too easy.

CONTENT

1. *Main and second main stroke*: from back crawl, front crawl and breast stroke.

2. *Other strokes*: side stroke, elementary back stroke and breast stroke kick in the supine position.

3. *New stroke*: butterfly dolphin or butterfly breast stroke.

4. *Part practices*: kicking and pulling.

5. *Open and spin turns*: on back crawl, front crawl and breast stroke.

6. *Other skills*: sculling, treading water and towing.

EXAMPLE WORKOUTS

1. Swimming workouts should take between 20 and 40 minutes.

2. Distances should only be increased after checking for distance improvement (see instructions).

WORKING INSTRUCTIONS

1. **Warm-up** – Prior to starting the swimming workout, do 5–10 minutes of body stretching activities on the pool side and in the water.

2. **Body joints** – Are you stretching and bending those joints?

3. **Pace** – Maintain a consistent pace and remember to swim the shorter distances at a faster pace than the longer ones.

4. **Rest** – Rest for up to $1\frac{1}{2}$ minutes between workout phases; you may find that you can adjust rest time according to the intensity of a phase and how you feel.

5. **Cool-down** – After the swimming workout, swim slowly for a few minutes and then do some body stretching on the pool side to reduce the heart rate and to avoid stiffness.

LEVEL II – EXAMPLES

EXAMPLE I

MAIN STROKE: Front crawl.
SECOND STROKE: Breast stroke.
DISTANCE: 600 metres.
OTHER SKILLS: Treading water.
EQUIPMENT: Float or kick board and pull buoy, clock or watch.

Phase	Practice	Focus
1. Full stroke	Swim 100 metres on FRONT CRAWL	Work hard from the hips in both the upwards and downwards movements
2. Part practice	Hold the float half-way along and extend the arms: kick 2 × 50 metres on FRONT CRAWL (rest for 35 seconds after the first 50 metres)	Initiate the kicking movements from the hips
3. Part practice	Place the float between the upper parts of the legs: pull 2 × 50 metres on FRONT CRAWL (rest for 30 seconds after the first 50 metres)	Recover the arms by lifting the elbows high over the water surface
4. Full stroke	Swim 100 metres on FRONT CRAWL	Recover with the elbows high and the hands low
5. Full stroke	Swim 100 metres on BREAST STROKE	Stretch the arms forwards beneath the water surface
6. Treading water	Water at shoulder level: tread water using the legs and one arm ($1\frac{1}{2}$ minutes) and tread water using the legs and the other arm ($1\frac{1}{2}$ minutes)	Bend at the knees and hook and turn the feet outwards as in the breast stroke kick; rotate the legs inwards and straighten
7. Full stroke	Swim 100 metres; alternate FRONT CRAWL and BREAST STROKE, changing after each 25 metres	Lead all propulsive arm movements with the hands

QUESTIONS

1. Did you keep the legs moving?
2. Did you ache in the upper parts of the legs?
3. Did you keep the elbows close to the face?
4. Are you getting your elbows higher?
5. Did you manage a short glide?
6. Can you feel the circular action?
7. Can you feel the pressure on your hands?

EXAMPLE 2

MAIN STROKE: Back crawl
SECOND STROKES: Side stroke, elementary back stroke, breast stroke kick in the supine position,
butterfly dolphin.
DISTANCE: 600 metres.
OTHER SKILLS: None.
EQUIPMENT: Float or pull buoy, clock or watch.

Phase	Practice	Focus
1. Full stroke	Swim 100 metres on BACK CRAWL	Pull to the side with a wide shallow straight arm movement or pull with a bent arm and push to a straight arm close to the body ('S' movement)
2. Full stroke	Swim 100 metres on 4 STROKES; swim 25 metres each on back crawl, side stroke, elementary back stroke and breast stroke kick in the supine position (scull with the hands) in any order	Maintain a firm wrist during all propulsive arm movements
3. Part practice	Place the float between the upper parts of the legs; pull 100 metres on BACK CRAWL	Accelerate the hands during the propulsive stage of the arm action
4. Full stroke	Swim 50 metres on ELEMENTARY BACK STROKE	Recover the arms beneath the water surface and close to the body to a 'Y' position beyond the head
5. Kicking	Shallow end: (i) hold the pool side and practise FRONT CRAWL kicking (3 sets of 15 seconds); (ii) hold the pool side and practise BUTTERFLY DOLPHIN kicking (3 sets of 15 seconds)	Initiate the leg action from the hips and kick upwards as well as downwards
6. Full stroke	Shallow end: practise 3 or 4 BUTTERFLY DOLPHIN kicks followed by a BUTTERFLY DOLPHIN arm action and GLIDE	Kick with the arms extended in front of the body and then pull and recover the arms back to the extended position
7. Full stroke	Swim 5 × 50 metres on BACK CRAWL (30 seconds rest between each 50 metres)	Recover the arms high, straight and close to the body line

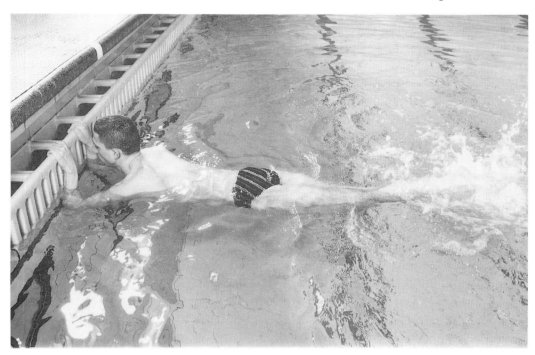

Front crawl kick using a bent-arm hold.

QUESTIONS

1. Did you move from the pull straight into the recovery?
2. Did you find it easy to change from one stroke to another?
3. Did you 'hold' the water?
4. Did you keep the hands beneath the water surface?
5. Did you concentrate on the upwards movement?
6. Did you manage a width on butterfly dolphin?
7. Did you brush the ears with the upper arms?

EXAMPLE 3

MAIN STROKE: Breast stroke.
SECOND STROKES: Front crawl, back crawl.
DISTANCE: 700 metres.
OTHER SKILLS: Breast stroke turn.
EQUIPMENT: Float or kick board and pull buoy, clock or watch.

Phase	Practice	Focus
1. Full stroke	Swim 100 metres; alternate FRONT CRAWL and BACK CRAWL changing after each 25 metres	Move the legs upwards and downwards in a rhythmic and regular action
2. Full stroke	Swim 8 × 25 metres on BREAST STROKE (rest for 15 seconds between each 25 metres)	Kick with the feet hooked and turned outwards
3. Part practice	Hold the float half-way along and extend the arms: kick 100 metres on BREAST STROKE	Kick backwards, outwards and together in vigorous and continuous movements
4. Turning	Shallow end: swim on BREAST STROKE to the pool side from a distance of 5 metres and practise an open turn (5 repetitions)	Touch the wall with two hands, turn and sink with the hands close to the head; stretch and glide away from the wall
5. Full stroke	Swim 2 × 50 metres on BREAST STROKE (rest for 30 seconds after the first 50 metres)	Stretch and glide away from the wall; surface by pulling the arms to the sides, gliding and then kicking and thrusting the arms forwards
6. Part practice	Place the float between the upper parts of the legs: pull 2 × 25 metres on BREAST STROKE (rest for 15 seconds after the first 25 metres)	Pause only for a moment with the arms in the extended recovery position
7. Full stroke	Swim 150 metres on 3 STROKES: swim 25 metres on back crawl, breast stroke, front crawl and then repeat	Swim with a steady and regular leg action on the crawl type strokes and a glide on the breast stroke

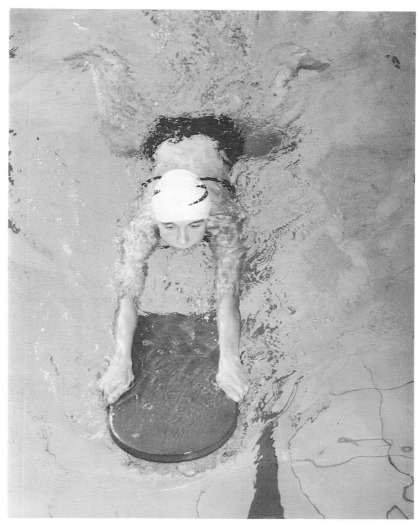

Breast stroke kick holding a kick board.

QUESTIONS

1. Did you keep the legs moving continuously?
2. Did you feel the surge forwards?
3. Did you turn the feet outwards just prior to the kick?
4. Did you turn and get a good glide?
5. Did you manage the complete turn?
6. Did you find this difficult?
7. Did you enjoy the medley swim?

EXAMPLE 4

SECOND MAIN STROKE: Own choice.
OTHER STROKES: Side stroke, elementary back stroke, breast stroke kick in the supine position, medley strokes.
DISTANCE: 700 metres.
OTHER SKILLS: Treading water, towing.
EQUIPMENT: Float or pull buoy, clock or watch.

Phase	Practice	Focus
1. Full stroke	Swim 100 metres on SIDE STROKE	Bend and spread the legs to recover; straighten and bring the legs together to kick
2. Treading water	Water at shoulder level: tread water using the legs and one arm (1½ minutes) and tread water using the legs and the other arm (1½ minutes)	Keep the head back and the face just clear of the water surface
3. Full stroke	Swim 100 metres on ELEMENTARY BACK STROKE	Sweep the arms round and to the sides from the 'Y' position beyond the head
4. Towing	Partner places the float between the upper parts of the legs: using a BREAST STROKE kick in the SUPINE position and one arm (sculling), tow your partner 2 × 25 metres by the CHIN TOW (rest for 15 seconds after the first 25 metres)	Hold the chin and keep the subject's head close to your shoulder
5. Full stroke	Swim 350 metres on your SECOND MAIN STROKE	Accelerate the hands in the propulsive arm movement and feel the water pressure on the palms of the hands
6. Full stroke	Swim 100 metres INDIVIDUAL MEDLEY (swim 25 metres each on butterfly dolphin or butterfly breast stroke, back crawl, breast stroke and front crawl)	Accelerate the hands in all propulsive arm movements

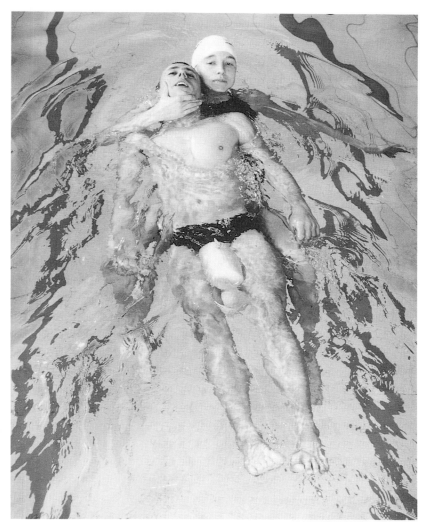

Chin tow with subject's legs supported by a pull buoy.

QUESTIONS

1. Did you stay on the side?
2. Did you feel in control?
3. Did you get the hands to the sides?
4. Did you keep your partner close to you?
5. Did you 'hold' the water?
6. Did you feel the surge forwards?

EXAMPLE 5

MAIN STROKE: Front crawl.
SECOND STROKES: Breast stroke, back crawl, butterfly dolphin or butterfly breast stroke.
DISTANCE: 800 metres.
OTHER SKILLS: None.
EQUIPMENT: Float or kick board and pull buoy, hand paddles, clock or watch.

Phase	Practice	Focus
1. Full stroke	Swim 100 metres on FRONT CRAWL	Exhale forcibly prior to taking a good inhalation
2. Part practice	Place the float between the upper parts of the legs: pull, using HAND PADDLES, 4 × 50 metres on FRONT CRAWL (rest for 30 seconds between each 50 metres)	Concentrate on keeping the elbows high during the first part of the arm propulsive movement
3. Full stroke	Swim 100 metres on FRONT CRAWL	Turn to the side of the arm that is completing the push stage; breathe to the same side every arm cycle
4. Part practice	Hold the float half-way along and extend the arms: kick 4 × 25 metres on FRONT CRAWL (rest for 20 seconds between each 25 metres)	Concentrate on kicking upwards from the hips
5. Full stroke	Swim 4 × 75 metres on 4 STROKES; swim 75 metres on breast stroke, 75 metres on back crawl, 75 metres on front crawl and 75 metres alternating butterfly dolphin, front crawl and back crawl every 25 metres (rest for 35 seconds between each 100 metres)	Lead all propulsive arm movements with the hands

QUESTIONS

1. Did you get a good breath?
2. Did you improve your 'hold' on the water?
3. Did you get into a breathing rhythm?
4. Did you keep the legs close to the water surface?
5. Did you get 'hold' of the water on all strokes?

EXAMPLE 6

MAIN STROKE: Back crawl.
SECOND STROKES: Butterfly dolphin or butterfly breast stroke, breast stroke, front crawl.
DISTANCE: 800 metres.
OTHER SKILLS: None.
EQUIPMENT: Float or kick board and pull buoy, hand paddles, clock or watch.

Phase	Practice	Focus
1. Full stroke	Swim 200 metres on BACK CRAWL	Keep the hips up and pillow the head on the water surface
2. Full stroke	Swim 8 × 25 metres on the 4 INDIVIDUAL MEDLEY STROKES; swim butterfly dolphin or butterfly breast stroke, back crawl, breast stroke and front crawl and repeat the sequence (rest for 15 seconds between each 25 metres)	Learn the individual medley order of butterfly dolphin, back crawl, breast stroke and front crawl
3. Part practice	Hold the float between the upper parts of the legs: pull, using HAND PADDLES, 100 metres on BACK CRAWL	Bend and straighten the arms during the up and down hand movements along the body

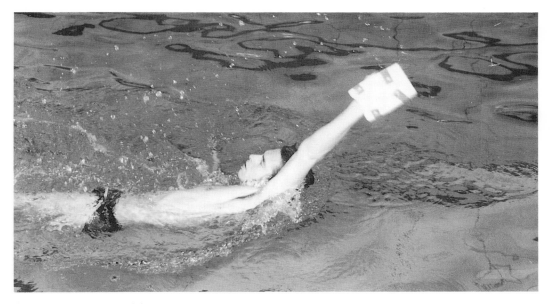

Back crawl using hand paddles.

Phase	Practice	Focus
4. Full stroke	Swim 100 metres on 3 STROKES; swim 25 metres on butterfly dolphin or butterfly breast stroke, 25 metres on breast stroke and 50 metres on front crawl	Control all recovery arm movements whether they are above or below the water surface
5. Part practice	Hold the float above the hips; kick 4 × 25 metres on BACK CRAWL (rest for 20 seconds between each 25 metres)	Extend the legs and force the toes to the water surface
6. Full stroke	Swim 100 metres on BACK CRAWL	Keep the hips up and just below the water surface

QUESTIONS

1. Did you maintain a streamlined body position close to the water surface?
2. Are you getting used to the individual medley order?
3. Did you get an effective pull?
4. Did you find that you could change easily from one stroke to another?
5. Did you keep the legs close to the water surface?
6. Did you keep the hips up?

EXAMPLE 7

MAIN STROKE: Breast stroke.
SECOND STROKE: Front crawl.
DISTANCE: 900 metres.
OTHER SKILLS: None.
EQUIPMENT: Float or kick board and pull buoy, hand paddles, clock or watch.

Phase	Practice	Focus
1. Full stroke	Swim 100 metres on BREAST STROKE	Sweep the legs round and together in a vigorous and continuous movement
2. Part practice	Hold the float half-way along and extend the arms (prone position) and hold the float above the hips (supine position): kick 200 metres on BREAST STROKE changing from the prone to the supine position after each 25 metres	Recover slowly and kick quickly
3. Full stroke	Swim 100 metres on BREAST STROKE	Keep the arm action in front of a line dropped from the shoulders
4. Part practice	Hold the float between the upper parts of the legs: pull, using HAND PADDLES, 2 × 50 metres on BREAST STROKE (rest for 30 seconds after the first 50 metres)	Pull and recover in a continuous action
5. Part practice	Swim 4 × 50 metres on FRONT CRAWL; on each 50 metres swim the first 25 metres using the legs and the left arm and the second 25 metres using the legs and the right arm (rest for 30 seconds between each 50 metres)	Recover the elbows high and point the fingers downwards in the early part of the movement
6. Full stroke	Swim 200 metres; alternate FRONT CRAWL and BREAST STROKE changing after each 25 metres	Accelerate the hands during the propulsive movements

QUESTIONS

1. Did you feel the pressure on the insides of the feet?
2. Did you surge forwards as you kicked?
3. Did the hands give you support?
4. Are the hands still giving you support?
5. Are you getting the elbows higher now?
6. Did you get an effective pull?

EXAMPLE 8

SECOND MAIN STROKE: Own choice.
OTHER STROKES: Butterfly dolphin or butterfly breast stroke, side stroke, elementary back
                 stroke.
DISTANCE: 900 metres.
OTHER SKILLS: Towing.
EQUIPMENT: Float or kick board and pull buoy, clock or watch.

Phase	Practice	Focus
1. Full stroke	Swim 150 metres on your SECOND MAIN STROKE	Kick continuously from the hips in the crawl type strokes; recover slowly and kick quickly in the breast stroke
2. Full stroke	Swim 4 × 25 metres on BUTTERFLY DOLPHIN or BUTTERFLY BREAST STROKE (rest for 40 seconds between each 25 metres)	Inhale just prior to the arm recovery
3. Full stroke	Swim 150 metres; alternate SIDE STROKE and ELEMENTARY BACK STROKE changing after each 25 metres	Keep the arm actions beneath the water surface
4. Towing	Partner places the float between the upper parts of the legs: using a BREAST STROKE kick in the SUPINE position and one arm (sculling), tow your partner 4 × 25 metres by the CHIN TOW (rest for 15 seconds after each 25 metres)	Maintain a firm chin hold and keep the subject's head close to your shoulder
5. Full stroke and part practice	Swim 4 × 50 metres on your SECOND MAIN STROKE; swim 50 metres, kick 50 metres, pull 50 metres, swim 50 metres (rest for 30 seconds between each 50 metres)	Maintain steady and regular limb actions
6. Full stroke	Swim 200 metres on 4 STROKES: swim 50 metres on your second main stroke, 25 metres on butterfly dolphin or butterfly breast stroke, 25 metres on elementary back stroke, 50 metres on side stroke and 50 metres on your second main stroke	Move continuously from the propulsive movements into the recovery position

QUESTIONS

1. Are you improving your kick?
2. Did you get a good inhalation?
3. Did you adjust to the different arm actions?
4. Did you keep the subject's face above the water surface?
5. Did you get into a rhythm?
6. Is your second main stroke improving?

EXAMPLE 9

MAIN STROKES: Front crawl, back crawl.
SECOND STROKES: Butterfly dolphin, breast stroke.
DISTANCE: 1000 metres.
OTHER SKILLS: None.
EQUIPMENT: Float or kick board, hand paddles, clock or watch.

Phase	Practice	Focus
1. Full stroke	Swim 200 metres; alternate FRONT CRAWL and BACK CRAWL changing after each 50 metres	Touch with one hand, spin in a tucked position, sink with the hands close to the head and push vigorously off the wall into a streamlined glide
2. Full stroke	Swim 6 × 50 metres, using HAND PADDLES; alternate FRONT CRAWL and BACK CRAWL changing after each 50 metres (rest for 30 seconds between each 50 metres)	Pull and push in a continuous movement
3. Part practice	Hold the float half-way along and extend the arms: kick 100 metres on FRONT CRAWL and BUTTERFLY DOLPHIN changing after each 25 metres	Keep all leg actions close to the water surface
4. Full stroke	Swim 4 × 25 metres on BUTTERFLY DOLPHIN (rest for 40 seconds between each 25 metres)	Drop the head and swing the arms low over the water surface
5. Part practice	Swim 200 metres on FRONT CRAWL and BACK CRAWL changing after each 50 metres; on each 50 metres swim the first 25 metres using the legs and the left arm and the second 25 metres using the legs and the right arm	Kick vigorously and continuously from the hips

Phase	Practice	Focus
6. Full stroke	Swim 100 metres INDIVIDUAL MEDLEY; swim 25 metres each on butterfly dolphin, back crawl, breast stroke and front crawl	Push away from the wall with the body, head and limbs all in line

QUESTIONS

1. Did you get a good push off?
2. Did you keep the hand paddles moving?
3. Did you keep the legs close to the water surface?
4. Did you recover the arms over the water surface?
5. Did you keep the legs moving?
6. Did you get a good glide?

EXAMPLE 10

MAIN STROKES: Butterfly dolphin, back crawl, breast stroke, front crawl.
DISTANCE: 1000 metres.
OTHER SKILLS: None.
EQUIPMENT: Float or kick board and pull buoy, clock or watch.

Phase	Practice	Focus
1. Full stroke	Swim 200 metres FRONT CRAWL	Recover the arms by lifting the elbows close to the body line
2. Full stroke	Swim 200 metres INDIVIDUAL MEDLEY (swim 25 metres each on butterfly dolphin, back crawl, breast stroke, front crawl and then repeat)	Keep the hands moving continuously during the propulsive actions
3. Part practice	Kick 200 metres INDIVIDUAL MEDLEY (kick 50 metres each on butterfly dolphin, back crawl, breast stroke and front crawl)	Kick vigorously from the hips in the crawl type strokes and forcefully extend and bring the legs together in the breast stroke
4. Part practice	Pull 200 metres INDIVIDUAL MEDLEY (pull 25 metres each on butterfly dolphin, back crawl, breast stroke, front crawl and then repeat)	Increase the speed of the hand movements during the propulsive stages
5. Full stroke	Swim 4 × 50 metres INDIVIDUAL MEDLEY; 50 metres each on butterfly dolphin, back crawl, breast stroke and front crawl (rest for 30 seconds between each 50 metres)	Concentrate on maintaining a regular stroke rhythm with a breath every arm cycle

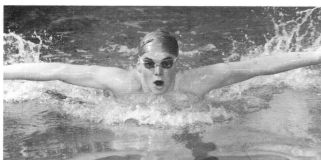

Individual medley stroke order:
a   Butterfly dolphin.

b   Back crawl.

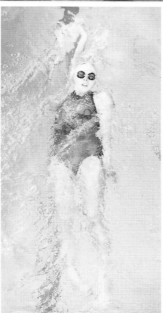

c   Breast stroke.

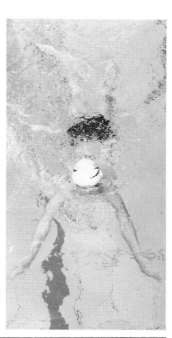

d   Front crawl.

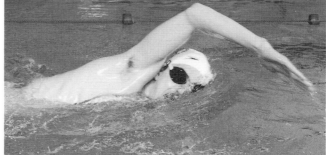

QUESTIONS

1. Are you feeling more mobile in the shoulders?
2. Did you lead all arm propulsive movements with the hands?
3. Did you kick hard?
4. Did you pull powerfully?
5. Are your strokes getting faster?

LEVEL III   (1100 METRES TO 1500 METRES)

How far do you want to go?

INSTRUCTIONS

1. You should only start on Level III if you have had experience of working through Level II.

2. From back crawl, front crawl and breast stroke, select your main stroke, your second main stroke and your third main stroke.

CONTENT

1. *Main, second and third main stroke*: from back crawl, front crawl and breast stroke.

2. *Other strokes*: butterfly dolphin, side stroke, elementary back stroke and breast stroke kick in the supine position.

3. *Part practices*: kicking and pulling.

4. *Open and spin turns*: on back crawl, front crawl and breast stroke.

5. *New turns*: back crawl spin turn with the head under and front crawl tumble turn.

6. *Other skills*: sculling and treading water.

7. *New skills*: plunge dive from the pool side and back stroke start.

EXAMPLE WORKOUTS

1. Swimming workouts should take between 30 and 50 minutes.

2. Start with workouts of 1100 metres and only increase the distance if you are finding the sessions comfortable and you are finishing well within or less than the allocated time for Level III workouts.

WORKING INSTRUCTIONS

1. **Warm-up** – This can be done in the form of some body stretching on the pool side and in the water but a swimming warm-up will now be included in each workout.

2. **Body joints** – Keep stretching and bending the joints.

3. **Pace** – You must place your own interpretation on the terms slow, moderate and fast.

4. **Rest** – Rest for 30 seconds to 1 minute between workout phases according to the intensity of a phase and how you feel.

5. **Cool-down** – A swimming cool-down to reduce the heart rate will now be included in each workout; and the body stretching, to avoid stiffness, will be done after completing the swimming workout.

TERMINOLOGY: LEVEL III

Training terms

The meaning of the terms has been adapted to suit the needs of the swimmers embarking on the progressive programme.

Overdistance training

Longer distances at slow and moderate paces, e.g. 400 metres over.

Fartlek training

Swimming, kicking and pulling any distance with pace variation.
Example – 200 metres: swim 25 metres slow and then 25 metres at a moderate pace and continue alternating until the 200 metres have been completed.

Interval training

Repeat swims over a stated distance (25 metres to 100 metres) at a given speed with a given rest time between each swim to allow partial recovery. By adjusting one of the four variables (i.e. number of repetitions, distance, speed and rest) the intensity of the workout can be increased. Kicking and pulling can also be organised in an interval training form.
Example – 6 × 50 metres, moderate pace, rest for 30 seconds between each repetition.

Specific terms

Some terms have been specifically applied to a type of training although they could be regarded as a form of interval training.

Negative split

The second half of the stated distance (50 metres to 100 metres) is swum at a faster pace than the first half.
Example – 4 × 50 metres: the second 25 metres is at least 2 seconds faster than the first 25 metres, rest for 30 seconds between each repetition.

Descending set (speed)

Repeat swims over a stated distance (50 metres to 100 metres) with the same rest time but with the speed increasing.
Example – 4 × 50 metres, increasing the speed from a moderate to fast pace (each repetition getting faster); rest for 25 seconds between each repetition.

Descending set (rest)

Repeat swims over a stated distance (50 metres to 100 metres) at a given speed with the rest being reduced with each repetition.
Example – 4 × 50 metres, fast pace; rest for 35 seconds after the first 50 metres, 30 seconds after the second 50 metres and 25 seconds after the third 50 metres.

Sprint training

Repeat swims over a short distance (25 metres to 50 metres) at a fast pace with a given rest time between each swim to allow a good recovery.
Example – 6 × 25 metres, fast pace, rest for 1 minute between each repetition.

Other terms

Bi-lateral

Breathe every third arm pull on front crawl to allow the swimmer to breathe on alternate sides.

Catch-up

Wait until the recovery arm catches up with the arm that is about to pull; there will be a pause with both arms extended in the front position (front crawl and back crawl).

LEVEL III – EXAMPLES

EXAMPLE 1

MAIN STROKE: Front crawl, back crawl.
DISTANCE: 1100 metres.
OTHER SKILLS: None.
EQUIPMENT: Float or kick board and pull buoy, clock or watch.

Phase/Pace	Practice	Focus
1. Warm-up, full stroke Slow	Swim 200 metres; alternate FRONT CRAWL and BACK CRAWL, changing after each 25 metres	Recover the arms high and close to the shoulder line
2. Part practice Moderate	Kick 150 metres; alternate FRONT CRAWL and BACK CRAWL, changing after each 25 metres	Concentrate on kicking upwards
3. Full stroke Slow and fast	Swim 200 metres on FRONT CRAWL; alternate slow and fast swims, changing the speed after each 25 metres	Pull and kick slowly on one length and pull and kick vigorously on the next length
4. Part practice Moderate	Pull 150 metres; alternate FRONT CRAWL and BACK CRAWL, changing after each 25 metres	Keep the fingers together and hold the wrists firm
5. Full stroke Fast	Swim 4 × 50 metres on BACK CRAWL; swim the second 25 metres of each 50 metres faster than the first (rest for 30 seconds between each 50 metres)	Speed up the stroke by accelerating the pulling action
6. Cool-down, full stroke Slow	Swim 200 metres; alternate FRONT CRAWL and BACK CRAWL, changing after 100 metres	Look upwards in back crawl and look forwards and downwards in the non-breathing phase of front crawl

QUESTIONS

1. Did you loosen up the shoulder joint?
2. Did you keep the legs moving?
3. Did you know that this is called FARTLEK training?
4. Did you 'hold' the water?
5. Did you know that this is a form of INTERVAL TRAINING called a NEGATIVE SPLIT?
6. Did you enjoy the workout?

EXAMPLE 2

MAIN STROKE: Breast stroke.
SECOND STROKES: Front crawl, back crawl.
DISTANCE: 1100 metres.
OTHER SKILLS: Plunge diving.
EQUIPMENT: Clock or watch.

Phase/Pace	Practice	Focus
1. Warm-up full stroke Slow	Swim 200 metres on 3 STROKES; swim 25 metres on front crawl, 25 metres on back crawl and 50 metres on breast stroke and then repeat	Keep the feet stretched on front crawl and back crawl; keep the feet hooked and turned outwards on breast stroke
2. Full stroke Moderate to fast	Pull 4 × 50 metres on BREAST STROKE; pull the first 50 metres at a moderate pace and swim faster with each succeeding 50 metres (rest for 25 seconds between each repetition)	Increase the speed of the pulling arm for greater speed
3. Diving	Deep water: practise a plunge dive (practise for 5 minutes)	Hold the arms behind the body, curl the toes round the pool side, bend the knees, round the back and bring the trunk forwards at the hips. Swing the arms forwards, overbalance and stretch from the fingertips to the toes
4. Full stroke Moderate	Dive and swim 4 × 50 metres on FRONT CRAWL (start in the deep end of the pool and rest for 40 seconds between each 50 metres)	Tense the body in flight and on entry
5. Full stroke Moderate	Swim 200 metres on BREAST STROKE	Extend the arms beneath the water surface and pause for a moment
6. Full stroke Slow and fast	Swim 200 metres FARTLEK on BREAST STROKE changing the speed after each 50 metres	Hold a longer glide on the slow 50 metres
7. Cool-down, full stroke Slow	Swim 100 metres; alternate BACK CRAWL and BREAST STROKE. changing after each 25 metres	Breathe every arm cycle

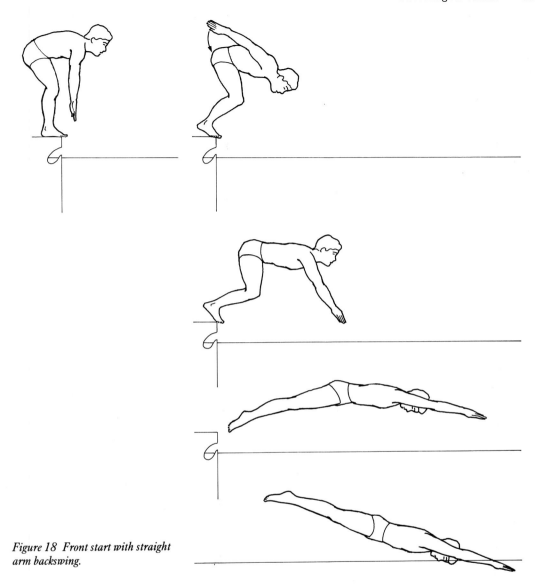

Figure 18 Front start with straight arm backswing.

QUESTIONS

1. Did you get the ankle position right?
2. (a) Did you check the times?
   (b) Did you know that this is a form of INTERVAL TRAINING called a DESCENDING SET (speed)?
3. Did you keep the arms stretched beyond the head?
4. Did you keep the body and limbs rigid on entry?
5. Did you manage a short glide?
6. Do you understand the term FARTLEK?
7. Are you recovering quickly?

EXAMPLE 3

MAIN STROKE: Back crawl.
SECOND STROKES: Butterfly dolphin, breast stroke, back crawl.
DISTANCE: 1200 metres.
OTHER SKILLS: Back crawl start.
EQUIPMENT: Float or kick board, clock or watch.

Phase/Pace	Practice	Focus
1. Warm-up, full stroke Slow	Swim 150 metres on 3 STROKES; swim 75 metres on breast stroke, 50 metres on front crawl and 25 metres on back crawl	Breathe every arm cycle and exhale forcibly before inhaling
2. Part practice Moderate	Swim 150 metres on BACK CRAWL; use the legs and the left arm for the first 25 metres, the legs and the right arm for the second 25 metres and then repeat	Pull and bend the arms and then push and straighten the arms ('S' movement)
3. Part practice Moderate	Kick 150 metres on BACK CRAWL; kick with the hands on the hips for the first 25 metres, kick with the hands sculling by the hips for the second 25 metres and then repeat	Straighten the legs on the upwards movement and force the extended toes to the water surface.
4. Starting	Water at shoulder level: practise the back stroke start (practise for 5 minutes)	Hug the side closely in a close tuck position and then explode backwards. Swing the arms round and together, take the head back and keep the hips up
5. Full stroke Moderate	Swim 8 × 50 metres on BACK CRAWL (rest for 30 seconds after the first 50 metres, 25 seconds after the second 50 metres and then repeat)	Recover the extended arms high over the water surface and keep the upper arms close to the ears
6. Part practice Moderate	Swim 8 × 25 metres on BUTTERFLY DOLPHIN; use the legs and the left arm for the first 25 metres, the legs and the right arm for the second 25 metres and then repeat (rest for 25 seconds between each 25 metres)	Keep kicking the extended toes to the water surface
7. Cool-down, full stroke Slow	Swim 150 metres on 3 STROKES; swim 50 metres each on breast stroke, back crawl and front crawl	Breathe every arm cycle on all strokes

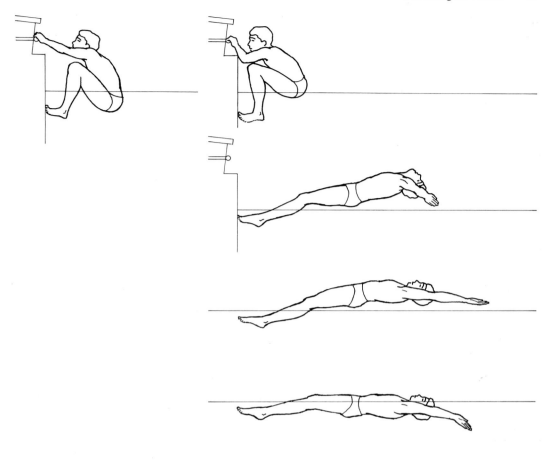

Figure 19 Back stroke start.

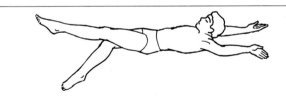

QUESTIONS

1. Did you get into a breathing rhythm?
2. Did you get the final push?
3. Did you keep a continuous leg action going close to the water surface?
4. Did you get a good arch?
5. Did you have control over the arm recovery?
6. Did you keep the leg action close to the water surface?
7. Are you still keeping up a breathing rhythm?

EXAMPLE 4

MAIN STROKE: Front crawl.
SECOND STROKES: Breast stroke, back crawl.
DISTANCE: 1200 metres.
OTHER SKILLS: None.
EQUIPMENT: Float or kick board and pull buoy, hand paddles, clock or watch.

Phase/Pace	Practice	Focus
1. Warm-up, full stroke Slow	Swim 150 metres; alternate BREAST STROKE and BACK CRAWL, changing after each 25 metres	Keep the wrists firm and the fingers together during the pull and push
2. Part practice Moderate	Pull, using HAND PADDLES, 150 metres on FRONT CRAWL	Keep the pulling action close to the centre line of the body

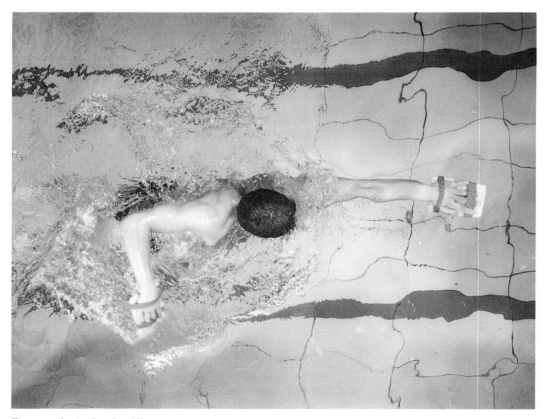

Front crawl using hand paddles.

Phase/Pace	Practice	Focus
3. Full stroke Fast	Swim 4 × 50 metres on FRONT CRAWL (rest for 35 seconds after the first 50 metres, 30 seconds after the second 50 metres and 25 seconds after the third 50 metres)	Concentrate on keeping the elbows high on the first part of the pull even when the rest time gets less
4. Part practice Slow and fast	Kick 150 metres FARTLEK on FRONT CRAWL, changing the speed after each 25 metres	Work more vigorously from the hips on the faster 25 metres
5. Full stroke Moderate	Swim 400 metres on FRONT CRAWL	Inhale to the side when the breathing-side arm is completing the push and the non-breathing-side arm has just entered the water
6. Cool-down, full stroke Slow	Swim 150 metres on 3 STROKES; swim 50 metres each on breast stroke, back crawl and front crawl	Breathe regularly every arm cycle

QUESTIONS

1. Did you 'hold' the water?
2. Did you feel the acceleration?
3. Did you know that this is a form of INTERVAL TRAINING called a DESCENDING SET (rest)?
4. Did you kick at varying speeds?
5. Did you turn the head smoothly?
6. Did you find this relaxing?

EXAMPLE 5

MAIN STROKES: Butterfly dolphin, back crawl, breast stroke, front crawl.
DISTANCE: 1300 metres.
OTHER SKILLS: None.
EQUIPMENT: Clock or watch.

Phase/Pace	Practice	Focus
1. Warm-up, full stroke and part practice Slow	Swim and kick 200 metres on 2 STROKES; swim 25 metres on front crawl, 25 metres on dog's paddle, 25 metres on back crawl, 25 metres on back crawl kick with the hands sculling by the hips and then repeat	Move the arms alternately, beneath the water surface and in front of the shoulders with dog's paddle
2. Full stroke Moderate	Swim 400 metres INDIVIDUAL MEDLEY (swim 25 metres each on butterfly dolphin, back crawl, breast stroke and front crawl and then repeat)	Touch two-handed after butterfly dolphin, one-handed after back crawl, two-handed after breast stroke and one-handed after front crawl
3. Part practice Moderate	Kick 200 metres INDIVIDUAL MEDLEY (kick 25 metres each on butterfly dolphin, back crawl, breast stroke and front crawl and then repeat)	Keep the feet stretched on the crawl type leg actions; keep the feet hooked and turned outwards on breast stroke
4. Full stroke and part practice Moderate	Swim and kick 200 metres on INDIVIDUAL MEDLEY; swim 25 metres on butterfly dolphin, kick 25 metres on butterfly dolphin with a breast stroke arm action, swim 25 metres on back crawl, kick 25 metres on back crawl with the hands sculling by the hips, swim 25 metres on breast stroke, kick 25 metres on breast stroke with the arms extended in front and the occasional breast stroke arm action, swim 25 metres on front crawl and 25 metres on dog's paddle	Lead all pulling movements with the hands; stretch the toes on the crawl type leg actions and hook and turn the feet outwards on breast stroke
5. Full stroke Fast	Swim 100 metres INDIVIDUAL MEDLEY (swim 25 metres each on butterfly dolphin, back crawl, breast stroke and front crawl)	Concentrate on getting a good exhalation before inhaling
6. Cool-down, full stroke Slow	Swim 200 metres on SECOND MAIN STROKE	Move the limbs slowly but at a speed that maintains a near horizontal position

QUESTIONS

1. Did you cope easily with all these adjustments?
2. Did you get the Individual Medley order correct?
3. Did you adjust your feet for the breast stroke kick?
4. Do you feel that you have control over the stroke movements?
5. Did you get into a breathing rhythm at this speed?
6. Did you recover during the swim?

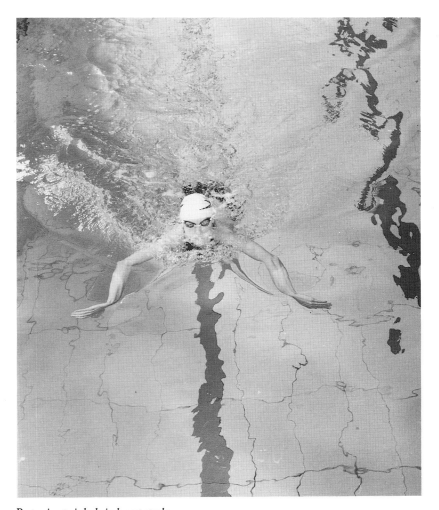

Preparing to inhale in breast stroke.

EXAMPLE 6

MAIN STROKE: Breast stroke.
SECOND STROKES: Elementary back stroke, side stroke, front crawl.
DISTANCE: 1300 metres.
OTHER SKILLS: None.
EQUIPMENT: Float or kick board and pull buoy, clock or watch.

Phase/Pace	Practice	Focus
1. Warm-up, full stroke Slow	Swim 200 metres on BREAST STROKE	Sweep the legs round and together in a vigorous and rapid movement
2. Full stroke Moderate	Swim 200 metres on ELEMENTARY BACK STROKE	Recover the arms beneath the water surface to the 'Y' position
3. Part practice Moderate	Pull 150 metres on BREAST STROKE	Keep the arms in front of the shoulders and pause briefly in the extended position
4. Full stroke Moderate	Swim 200 metres on SIDE STROKE	Spread and bend the legs on the recovery and bring together and straighten on the kick
5. Part practice Moderate	Kick 150 metres on BREAST STROKE	Accelerate the legs during the kick
6. Full stroke Fast	Swim 4 × 50 metres on BREAST STROKE (rest for 30 seconds between each 50 metres)	Pull and recover in a continuous action
7. Cool-down, full stroke Slow	Swim 200 metres; alternate back crawl and front crawl changing after each 50 metres	Look upwards in back crawl; look forwards and downwards in the non-breathing stage of front crawl; look sideways and forwards in the breathing stage of the front crawl

QUESTIONS

1. Did you feel the acceleration as you kicked?
2. Did you get the timing right?
3. Did you find this tiring?
4. Did you feel the acceleration as you kicked?
5. Did you feel the power in your legs?
6. Did you work the arms in front of the shoulders?
7. Did you get the head position right?

EXAMPLE 7

MAIN STROKE: Breast stroke.
SECOND STROKES: Butterfly dolphin, back crawl, front crawl.
DISTANCE: 1400 metres.
OTHER SKILLS: Breast stroke turn.
EQUIPMENT: Hand paddles, clock or watch.

Phase/Pace	Practice	Focus
1. Warm-up, full stroke Slow	Swim 200 metres on BREAST STROKE	Recover the legs by trying to get the heels close to the buttocks
2. Turning	Water at shoulder level: swim on BREAST STROKE to the pool side from a distance of 5 metres and practise an open turn (practise for 5 minutes)	Turn, sink and bring the hands to a position close to the head. Stretch and glide away from the wall, pull to the sides and glide, kick and stretch the arms to the water surface

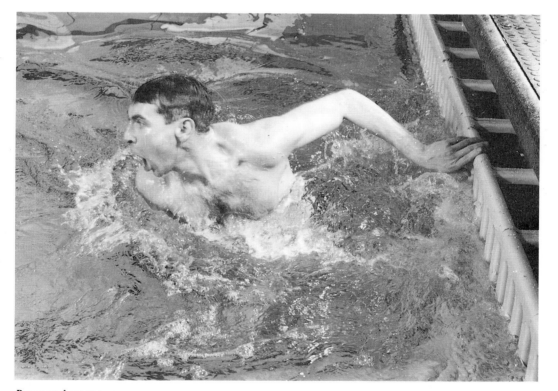

Breast stroke open turn.

Phase/Pace	Practice	Focus
3. Full stroke and part practice Moderate	Swim, kick and pull 400 metres on BREAST STROKE; swim 100 metres on breast stroke, kick 100 metres on breast stroke with the arms extended in front and the occasional breast stroke arm action, pull 100 metres on breast stroke using a dolphin kick and swim 100 metres breast stroke	Glide briefly with the arms extended during the full stroke and kicking practices and pause for a short moment with the arms extended in the pulling practice
4. Part practice Slow and moderate	Pull, using HAND PADDLES, 200 metres FARTLEK, on BREAST STROKE, changing the speed after each 25 metres	Accelerate the paddles more on the moderate 25 metres
5. Full stroke Moderate	Swim 200 metres INDIVIDUAL MEDLEY (swim 50 metres each on butterfly dolphin, back crawl stroke and front crawl)	Swim the butterfly dolphin with a two beat leg kick and a brief arm glide
6. Full stroke Faster than usual	Swim 8 × 25 metres on BREAST STROKE (rest for 40 seconds between each 25 metres)	Pause for only a moment when the arms are extended
7. Cool-down, full stroke Slow	Swim 200 metres on FRONT CRAWL	Turn to the side of the arm that is completing the push and exhale forcibly before inhaling

QUESTIONS

1. Did you get the heels close to the seat?
2. Did you get the timing right?
3. Did you find this tiring?
4. Did you manage to change the speed of the arm action?
5. Did you manage the 50 metres on butterfly dolphin?
6. Did you know that this is a form of SPRINT TRAINING? (unlike interval training there is more time to recover before the next repetition)
7. Did you get an effective inhalation?

EXAMPLE 8

MAIN STROKE: Front crawl.
SECOND STROKE: Own choice.
DISTANCE: 1400 metres.
OTHER SKILLS: Tumble turn.
EQUIPMENT: Float or kick board and pull buoy, clock or watch.

Phase/Pace	Practice	Focus
1. Warm-up, full stroke Slow	Swim 200 metres on FRONT CRAWL	Concentrate on a forceful exhalation before inhalation
2. Full stroke Moderate	Swim 6 × 50 metres on FRONT CRAWL (rest for 30 seconds between each 50 metres)	Breathe on alternate sides by breathing every third arm pull
3. Turning	Water at shoulder level: (a) Practise forward somersaults away from the pool side (b) Practise forward somersaults about a metre from the pool side (c) Swim on FRONT CRAWL to the pool side from a distance of 5 metres and practise a forward somersault about a metre from the pool side and push off on the back (d) Swim on FRONT CRAWL to the pool side from a distance of 5 metres and practise a forward somersault about a metre from the pool side, push off on the back and twist on to the front	Pull the leading arm back to the body and force the head down and back; pike the body at the hips and bend the legs in a loose tuck. As the feet are brought over and placed against the wall, move the hands to a position beyond the head. Stretch away from the wall on to the front
4. Part practice Moderate	Pull 3 × 100 metres on FRONT CRAWL (rest for 40 seconds between each 100 metres)	Push the hands back to the hips in the final stage of the underwater movement
5. Full stroke Moderate	Swim 4 × 75 metres on FRONT CRAWL (rest for 35 seconds after the first 75 metres, 30 seconds after the second 75 metres and 25 seconds after the third 75 metres)	Concentrate on keeping the elbows high on the first part of the pull and then pushing the hands back to the hips in the final part even when the rest gets less
6. Part practice Moderate and fast	Kick 100 metres FARTLEK on FRONT CRAWL	Kick with the legs close together

7. Cool-down, full stroke Slow	Swim 200 metres on THIRD MAIN STROKE (if the stroke is front crawl select your second main stroke)	Maintain a steady limb action and breathe regularly

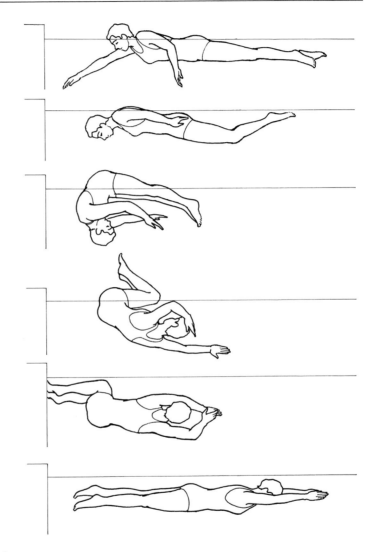

Figure 20 Front crawl tumble turn.

QUESTIONS

1. Did you get a good inhalation?
2. Did you know that this is called BI-LATERAL BREATHING?
3. (a) Did you manage a tumble turn?
   (b) Did you know that you can touch the wall with the feet only?
4. Did you get a long underwater movement?
5. Did you manage the DESCENDING SET (rest)?
6. Did you feel the feet brushing each other?
7. Did you recover during the swim?

EXAMPLE 9

MAIN STROKE: Front crawl.
SECOND STROKES: Back crawl, elementary back stroke, breast stroke kick in the supine position.
DISTANCE: 1500 metres.
OTHER SKILLS: None.
EQUIPMENT: Clock or watch.

Phase/Pace	Practice	Focus
1. Warm-up, full stroke Slow	Swim 200 metres on 2 STROKES; alternate ELEMENTARY BACK STROKE and BREAST STROKE KICK in the SUPINE position, changing after each 25 metres	Kick with the feet turned outwards and feel the pressure on the insides of the feet and lower legs
2. Full stroke Moderate	Swim 400 metres OVERDISTANCE TRAINING on FRONT CRAWL, using a CATCH-UP STROKE	Pause for a moment with both arms in front and extended – you will have to use the legs effectively!
3. Full stroke Slow and moderate	Swim 300 metres FARTLEK on FRONT CRAWL, changing the speed after each 25 metres	Change the pace from slow to moderate by speeding up the arm recovery
4. Full stroke Moderate	Swim 4 × 50 metres INTERVAL TRAINING on FRONT CRAWL (rest for 25 seconds between each 50 metres)	Keep the pulling action close to the centre line of the body with the palms facing mainly backwards
5. Full stroke Faster than usual	Swim 4 × 25 metres SPRINT TRAINING on FRONT CRAWL (rest for 40 seconds between each 25 metres)	Concentrate on a continuous hand push and arm recovery
6. Full stroke All out	Swim 2 × 25 metres SPRINT TRAINING on FRONT CRAWL (rest for 1 minute after the first 25 metres)	Concentrate on a continuous hand push and arm recovery and a continuous hand entry and pull
7. Cool-down, full stroke Slow	Swim 250 metres on BACK CRAWL	Keep the hips close to the water surface and look upwards

QUESTIONS

1. Did you get the feet turned out before the kick?
2. Did you keep the legs moving continuously?
3. Are you finding it easier to change the pace?
4. Did you keep the palms moving backwards?
5. Did you hold a fast pace?
6. Did you go all out or just fast?
7. Did you maintain a streamlined body position?

EXAMPLE 10

MAIN STROKE: Back crawl.
SECOND STROKES: Side stroke, elementary back stroke, breast stroke kick in the supine position.
DISTANCE: 1500 metres.
OTHER SKILLS: Back stroke turn.
EQUIPMENT: Float or kick board and pull buoy, watch or clock.

Phase/Pace	Practice	Focus
1. Warm-up, full stroke Slow	Swim 200 metres on 3 STROKES; swim 100 metres on side stroke, 50 metres on elementary back stroke and 50 metres on breast stroke kick in the supine position	With elementary back stroke, pull and kick; with side stroke, scissor and part the arms; with breast stroke kick in the supine position, kick by circling the legs towards each other
2. Turning	Water at shoulder level: swim on BACK CRAWL to the pool side from a distance of 5 metres and practise a head under spin turn (practise for 5 minutes)	Touch the wall with the palm of the hand and with the fingers pointing downwards and slightly inwards; bend the arm, take the head back and lift the legs round and over the water surface
3. Part practice Moderate	Pull 300 metres BACK CRAWL	Accelerate the hands through the pull and push stages of the 'S' movement
4. Part practice Moderate	Kick 200 metres BACK CRAWL	Work hard from the hips and straighten the legs at the end of the upwards movement
5. Full stroke Moderate	Swim 300 metres on BACK CRAWL	Bend and straighten the arms and keep close to the body ('S' movement)
6. Cool-down, full stroke and treading water Slow and tread water with minimum effort	Swim 250 metres on FRONT CRAWL, tread water for 3 minutes and swim 250 metres on BACK CRAWL (start in deep water)	Look forwards and downwards in the non-breathing stage of the front crawl, look upwards in both the back crawl and treading water movements

QUESTIONS

1. Are you improving on these strokes?
2. Did you get the legs out of the water?
3. Did you feel the water pressure on the hands?
4. Did you keep those knees under?
5. Did you 'hold' the water with the hands?
6. Were you in control of the various head positions?

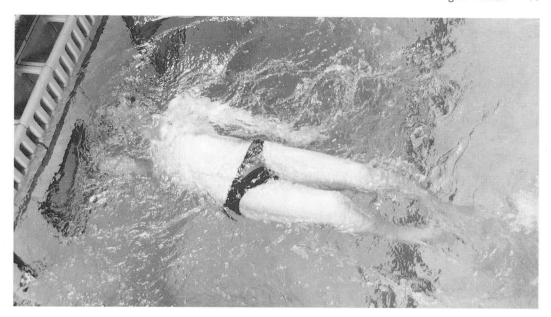

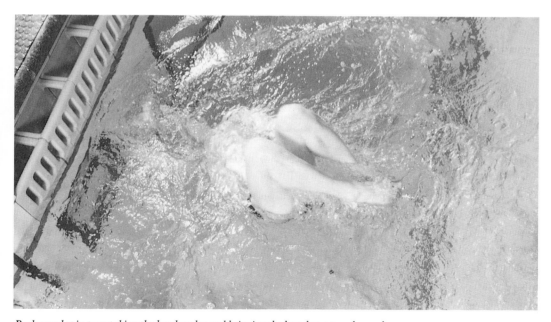

Back crawl spin turn taking the head under and bringing the bent legs up and round.

LEVEL IV (1600 METRES TO 2000 METRES)

Do you want to train on a regular basis?

INSTRUCTIONS

1. You should only start on Level IV if you have had experience of working through Level III.

2. From back crawl, front crawl and breast stroke, select your main stroke, your second main stroke and your third main stroke.

CONTENT

1. *Main, second and third stroke*: from back crawl, front crawl and breast stroke.

2. *Other strokes*: butterfly dolphin, side stroke, elementary back stroke and breast stroke kick in the supine position.

3. *New strokes*: inverted breast stroke, 'Old English' back stroke and trudgeon stroke.

4. *Part practices*: kicking and pulling.

5. *Open and spin turns*: on back crawl, front crawl, breast stroke and butterfly dolphin.

6. *Advanced turns*: front crawl tumble turn and back crawl spin turn with the head under.

7. *Other skills*: sculling, treading water, towing, plunge dive from the pool side and back stroke start.

8. *New skills*: surface diving.

9. *Other activities*: swimming with a partner and ball skills with a partner.

EXAMPLE WORKOUTS

1. Swimming workouts should take between 40 and 60 minutes.

2. Start with workouts of 1600 metres and only increase the distance if you are finding the sessions comfortable and you are finishing well within or less than the allocated time for Level IV workouts.

WORKING INSTRUCTIONS

1. **Warm-up** – This can be done in the form of some body stretching on the pool side and in the water, but a swimming warm-up will be included in each workout.

2. **Body joints** – Your general mobility should have improved but keep stretching and bending the joints.

3. **Pace** – Place your own interpretation on the terms slow, moderate and fast, but you will find that some repeat swims are controlled by time, e.g. 4×50 metres on 1 minute.

4. **Rest** – Rest for 30 seconds to 1 minute between workout phases according to the intensity of a phase and how you feel.

5. **Cool-down** – A swimming cool-down to reduce heart rate is included in each workout; and the body stretching, to avoid stiffness, will be done after completing the swimming workout.

TERMINOLOGY: LEVEL IV

Training terms	The meaning of the terms has been adapted to suit the needs of the swimmers embarking on the progressive programme.
Overdistance training	Longer distances at slow and moderate paces, e.g. 400 metres and over.

Fartlek training	Swimming, kicking and pulling any distance with pace variation. *Example* – 300 metres: swim 25 metres slow and then 25 metres at a fast pace and continue alternating until the 300 metres have been completed.
Interval training	Repeat swims over a stated distance (25 metres to 200 metres) at a given speed with a given rest time between each swim to allow partial recovery. By adjusting one of the four variables (i.e. number of repetitions, distance, speed and rest) the intensity of the workout can be increased. Kicking and pulling can also be organised in an interval training form. *Example* – 8 × 25 metres on 35 seconds (i.e. going every 35 seconds).
Sprint training	Repeat swims over a short distance (25 metres to 50 metres) at a fast pace with a given rest time between each swim to allow a good recovery. *Example* – 2 × 50 metres, fast pace, rest for 1 minute after the first 50 metres.

Specific terms

Some terms have been specifically applied to a type of training although they could be regarded as a form of interval training.

Negative split	The second half of the stated distance (50 metres to 200 metres) is swum at a faster pace than the first half. *Example* – 6 × 50 metres on 1 minute: the second 25 metres is faster than the first 25 metres.
Descending set (speed)	Repeat swims over a stated distance (50 metres to 200 metres) with the same rest time but with the speed increasing. *Example* – 3 × 50 metres on 1 minute, increasing the speed from a moderate to fast pace (each repetition getting faster).
Descending set (rest)	Repeat swims over a stated distance (50 metres to 200 metres) at a given speed with the rest being reduced with each repetition. *Example* – 10 × 25 metres, fast pace; go on for 40 seconds for swims 1, 2 and 3; on 35 seconds for swims 4, 5 and 6; and on 30 seconds for swims 7, 8 and 9.

Broken-swim   All-out repeat swims over short distances with very little rest, e.g. 4×25 metres, all out, rest for 5 seconds between each repetition.

Other terms

Bi-lateral   Breathe every third arm pull on front crawl to allow the swimmer to breathe on alternate sides.

Catch-up   Wait until the recovery arm catches up with the arm that is about to pull; there will be a pause with both arms extended in the front position (front crawl and back crawl).

LEVEL IV — EXAMPLES

EXAMPLE I

MAIN STROKE: Back crawl.
SECOND STROKES: Breast stroke, front crawl.
DISTANCE: 1600 metres.
OTHER SKILLS: None.
EQUIPMENT: Hand paddles, wrist weights, float or pull buoy, clock or watch.

Phase/Pace	Practice	Focus
1. Warm-up, full stroke Slow	Swim 150 metres on 3 STROKES; 50 metres each on back crawl, breast stroke and front crawl	Breathe every arm cycle at the same point in the arm stroke
2. Part practice Moderate	Kick 200 metres on BACK CRAWL; kick with the arms extended beyond the head for the first 25 metres, kick with the hands on the hips for the second 25 metres and then repeat	Turn the feet slightly inwards as the toes are forced to the water surface
3. Full stroke All out	Swim 4 × 25 metres on BACK CRAWL (5 seconds rest between each 25 metres	Be prepared to sink and stretch away from the wall after 5 seconds
4. Part practice Moderate	Pull, using HAND PADDLES, 200 metres on BACK CRAWL	Concentrate on establishing a regular and steady rhythm
5. Full stroke Fast	Swim 4 × 25 metres INTERVAL on BACK CRAWL on 40 seconds (i.e. you must go every 40 seconds)	Go every 40 seconds irrespective of the time taken for each 25 metres
6. Full stroke Moderate	Swim using WRIST WEIGHTS, 300 metres on BACK CRAWL	Recover sharply from the shoulders with straight arms
7. Full stroke Moderate	Swim 400 metres OVERDISTANCE on FRONT CRAWL	Establish a regular arm pattern and breathe every arm cycle at the same point in the arm stroke
8. Cool-down, full stroke Slow	Swim 150 metres on 3 STROKES; 50 metres each on back crawl, breast stroke and front crawl	Establish a regular arm pattern and keep the stroke alterations to the minimum on breathing

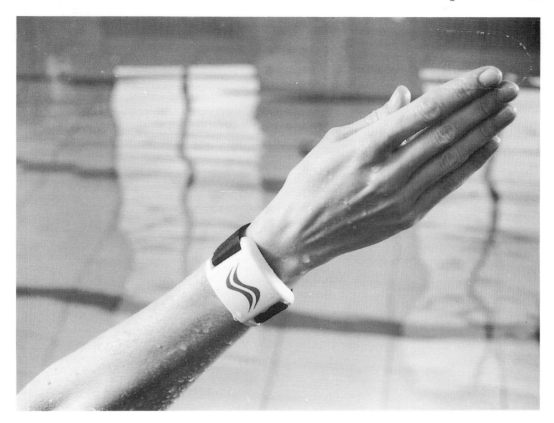

Wrist weight.

QUESTIONS

1. Did you get into a breathing rhythm?
2. Did you manage the practice with the arms extended beyond the head?
3. Did you know that this is called a BROKEN-SWIM?
4. Did you maintain a constant speed?
5. Did you follow the instructions by going every 40 seconds?
6. What difference did the weights make?
7. Did you breathe effectively every stroke cycle?
8. Did you maintain a breathing rhythm?

EXAMPLE 2

MAIN STROKE: Front crawl.
SECOND STROKE: Butterfly dolphin.
DISTANCE: 1600 metres.
OTHER SKILLS: None.
EQUIPMENT: Float or kick board and pull buoy, hand paddles, clock or watch.

Phase/Pace	Practice	Focus
1. Warm-up, full stroke Slow	Swim 150 metres CATCH-UP on FRONT CRAWL	Pause with both arms in front in an extended position with the hands touching
2. Full stroke Fast	Swim 4 × 50 metres INTERVAL on FRONT CRAWL on 1 minute 10 seconds	Keep the propulsive arm action as close to the body centre line as possible
3. Part practice Moderate	Kick 200 metres on FRONT CRAWL	Work the legs close to the water surface in a shallow movement
4. Full stroke Fast	Swim 8 × 25 metres INTERVAL on FRONT CRAWL on 35 seconds	Concentrate on a vigorous propulsive arm movement
5. Part practice Moderate	Pull 200 metres on FRONT CRAWL	Concentrate on lifting the elbows high enough at the start of the recovery to clear the water surface with the fingers
6. Full stroke Moderate	Swim, using HAND PADDLES, 200 metres on FRONT CRAWL	Lifting the paddles over the water surface can be helped with a shoulder roll
7. Full stroke Moderate	Swim 4 × 25 metres INTERVAL on BUTTERFLY DOLPHIN (rest for 15 seconds between each 25 metres)	Force the chin forwards as the arms are completing the push and about to recover
8. Full stroke Moderate	Swim 50 metres on BUTTERFLY DOLPHIN	Drop the face into the water and swing the arms low and round after the inhalation
9. Full stroke Moderate	Swim 150 metres on FRONT CRAWL; use the legs and the left arm for the first 25 metres, the legs and the right arm for the second 25 metres and then repeat	Maintain a moderate leg speed
10. Cool-down, full stroke Slow	Swim 150 metres on FRONT CRAWL	Recover the arms by lifting and bending; enter cleanly through the fingertips with the arms almost straight

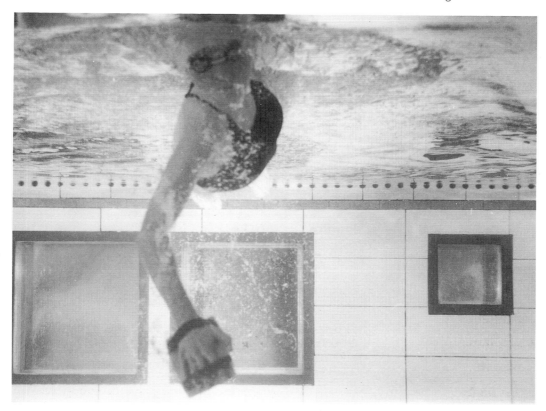

Front crawl using hand paddles and showing shoulder roll.

QUESTIONS

1. Did you stay relaxed with the catch-up stroke?
2. Did you keep to the time?
3. Did you keep the legs close to the water surface?
4. Did you keep to the time?
5. Did you get the elbows high?
6. Did you clear the water surface with the hand paddles?
7. Did you get the mouth clear of the water?
8. Did you get the head down?
9. Did you get the support from the legs?
10. Did you relax?

EXAMPLE 3

MAIN STROKES: Back crawl, breast stroke, front crawl.
SECOND STROKES: Inverted breast stroke, 'Old English' back stroke, side stroke, elementary back
stroke, butterfly dolphin.
DISTANCE: 1700 metres.
OTHER SKILLS: None.
EQUIPMENT: Clock or watch.

Phase/Pace	Practice	Focus
1. Warm-up, full stroke Slow	Swim 150 metres on 4 STROKES; select your own strokes and distances	Stretch as many joints as possible
2. Full stroke Moderate	Swim 4 × 100 metres INTERVAL on MAIN STROKE (rest for 35 seconds between each 100 metres)	Establish a breathing pattern
3. Full stroke Slow and fast	Swim 300 metres FARTLEK on SECOND MAIN STROKE, changing the speed after each 25 metres	Sharpen up the recovery and be more vigorous with the propulsive movement for the fast 25 metres
4. Full stroke Moderate	Swim 200 metres on THIRD MAIN STROKE	Concentrate on maintaining regular limb and breathing movements
5. Full stroke Moderate	Swim 100 metres on INVERTED BREAST STROKE	Sweep the straight arms round and to the sides from an extended position beyond the head and beneath the water surface; recover the legs and recover the arms simultaneously beneath the water surface to the extended position beyond the head. Kick as the arms move into the extended position
6. Full stroke Moderate	Swim 100 metres on 'OLD ENGLISH' BACK STROKE	Recover the legs (breast stroke leg movement) and recover the straight arms simultaneously high over the water surface to a position beyond the head. Pull and kick together
7. Full stroke Moderate	Swim 100 metres; alternate SIDE STROKE and ELEMENTARY BACK STROKE, changing after each 25 metres	Concentrate on the timing

Phase/Pace	Practice	Focus
8. Full stroke Moderate	Swim 200 metres INDIVIDUAL MEDLEY; swim 25 metres on each stroke and then repeat	Butterfly dolphin, back crawl, breast stroke and front crawl is the medley order
9. Cool-down, full stroke Slow	Swim 150 metres on OWN CHOICE STROKE	Maintain a slow steady rhythm in a near horizontal position

QUESTIONS

1. Did you feel the joints loosening up?
2. Did you get a good inhalation?
3. Did you manage the change of speed all the way?
4. Are you improving this stroke?
5. Did you get the timing right?
6. (a) Did you get the pull and kick together?
   (b) Did you find that you completed the leg kick before completing the arm pull?
7. Did you adjust easily to these strokes?
8. Did you remember the medley order?
9. Did you find a relaxing stroke?

EXAMPLE 4

MAIN STROKE: Breast stroke.
SECOND STROKES: Back crawl, front crawl, butterfly dolphin.
DISTANCE: 1700 metres.
OTHER SKILLS: None.
EQUIPMENT: Drag suit, float or kick board and pull buoy, clock or watch.

Phase/Pace	Practice	Focus
1. Warm-up, full stroke Slow	Swim 150 metres; organise in any way as long as you total 75 metres each on BACK CRAWL and FRONT CRAWL	Kick regularly and keep the legs close to the water surface
2. Full stroke Moderate	Swim, using a DRAG SUIT, 200 metres on BREAST STROKE	Glide briefly with the arms extended in front of the body

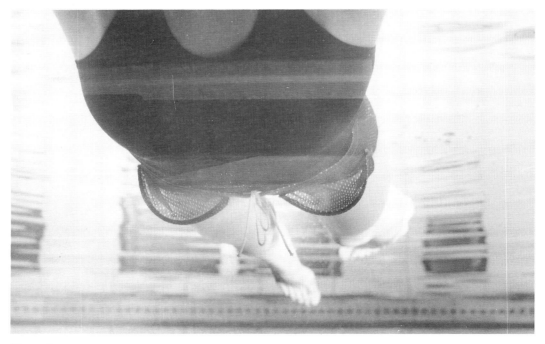

Drag suit.

Phase/Pace	Practice	Focus
3. Part practice Moderate	Pull 8 × 25 metres INTERVAL on BREAST STROKE on 1 minute	Breathe late in the arm pull and quickly recover the arms back to the extended position in front of the body
4. Part practice Moderate	Kick 6 × 50 metres INTERVAL on BREAST STROKE on 1 minute 30 seconds	Bend the legs and bring the heels close to the buttocks in preparation for the kick
5. Full stroke Moderate	Swim 4 × 100 metres INTERVAL on BREAST STROKE (rest for 35 seconds between each 100 metres)	Recover the arms quickly and kick when the arms are almost in the extended position in front of the body
6. Part practice Moderate	Swim 200 metres on BUTTERFLY DOLPHIN; use the legs and left arm for the first 25 metres, the legs and the right arm for the second 25 metres and then repeat	Initiate the leg movements from the hips and concentrate on the kick upwards
7. Full stroke Fast	Swim 2 × 50 metres SPRINT on BREAST STROKE (rest for 1 minute after the first 50 metres)	Pause only momentarily with the arms extended in front of the body
8. Cool-down, full stroke Slow	Swim 150 metres; alternate BACK CRAWL and FRONT CRAWL, changing after 75 metres	Rotate the arms slightly inwards during the propulsive actions

QUESTIONS

1. Did you kick steadily throughout the swim?
2. Did you maintain a constant pace?
3. Did you keep the arms moving?
4. Did you get a good recovery?
5. Did you get into an easy rhythym?
6. Did you get a good kick upwards?
7. Did you get into a fast rhythm?
8. Did you get the hands leading?

EXAMPLE 5

MAIN STROKE: Back crawl.
SECOND STROKES: Side stroke, elementary back stroke, trudgeon stroke.
DISTANCE: 1800 metres.
OTHER SKILLS: None.
EQUIPMENT: Drag ring, float or pull buoy, clock or watch.

Phase/Pace	Practice	Focus
1. Warm-up, full stroke Slow	Swim 200 metres; alternate SIDE STROKE and ELEMENTARY BACK STROKE, changing after each 50 metres	Glide on the side stroke after bringing the legs together and spreading the arms backwards and forwards; glide on the elementary back stroke after circling the legs towards each other and pulling the arms to the sides
2. Full stroke Moderate	Swim 2 × 200 metres INTERVAL on BACK CRAWL (rest for 1 minute 20 seconds after the first 200 metres)	Enter through the fingertips with the palms facing outwards
3. Full stroke Fast	Swim 4 × 50 metres INTERVAL on BACK CRAWL on 1 minute *or* 1 minute 10 seconds	Complete the push stage and immediately lift the straight arms out of the water with the palms facing inwards
4. Part practice Moderate	Pull and kick 200 metres on BACK CRAWL; kick 100 metres with the arms extended beyond the head-rest for 10 seconds – pull 100 metres	Enter cleanly through the fingertips and work the feet vigorously and close to the water surface
5. Full stroke Fast	Swim 8 × 25 metres INTERVAL on BACK CRAWL on 30 *or* 35 seconds	Complete the push stage and lift the straight arms sharply from the water
6. Full stroke All-out	Swim 4 × 25 metres BROKEN-SWIM on BACK CRAWL (5 seconds rest between each 25 metres)	Maintain a fast, controlled high recovery
7. Part practice Moderate	Pull, using a DRAG RING, 200 metres on FRONT CRAWL; use a pull buoy as well if the practice is too difficult	Concentrate on a continuous arm action

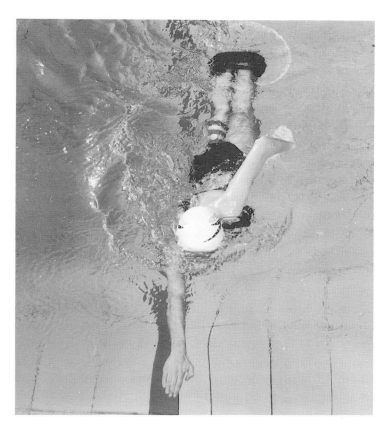

Front crawl pull using drag ring and supported by a pull buoy.

Phase/Pace	Practice	Focus
8. Full stroke Moderate	Swim 100 metres on TRUDGEON STROKE	Try either a side stroke or breast stroke leg action with a front crawl arm action
9. Cool-down, full stroke Slow	Swim 200 metres on BACK CRAWL	Keep the hips close to the water surface

QUESTIONS

1. Did you get an effective glide?
2. Did you feel as though you entered cleanly?
3. Did you keep the arms moving continuously?
4. Did you make the change within 10 seconds?
5. Did you get into a fast arm rhythm?
6. Did you go faster than the swim in phase 5?
7. Did you feel the drag?
8. Did you still breathe to the side?
9. Did you keep in a horizontal position?

EXAMPLE 6

MAIN STROKE: Front crawl.
SECOND STROKE: Butterfly dolphin.
DISTANCE: 1800 metres.
OTHER SKILLS: None.
EQUIPMENT: Training tube, drag belt, float or kick board, clock or watch.

Phase/Pace	Practice	Focus
1. Warm-up, full stroke Slow	Swim 150 metres on FRONT CRAWL	Enter through the fingertips; the arms are very slightly bent and the elbows are slightly higher than the hands
2. Full stroke Slow and moderate	Swim 200 metres FARTLEK on FRONT CRAWL; alternate slow and moderate swims, changing the speed after each 50 metres	Keep the palms moving mainly in the backwards direction in the propulsive stage
3. Full stroke Moderate	Pull, using a TRAINING TUBE, 250 metres on FRONT CRAWL	Keep the palms moving mainly backwards and close to the body centre line in the propulsive stage

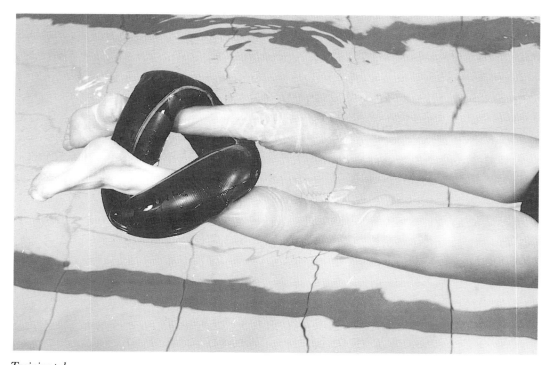

Training tube.

Phase/Pace	Practice	Focus
4. Full stroke Fast	Swim 6 × 50 metres NEGATIVE SPLIT on FRONT CRAWL on 55 seconds *or* I minute	Speed up both the legs and the arms on the second 25 metres
5. Full stroke Fast	Swim 10 × 25 metres DESCENDING SET (REST) on FRONT CRAWL; go on 40 seconds for swims I, 2 and 3, on 35 seconds for swims 4, 5 and 6, and on 30 seconds for swims 7, 8 and 9	Keep the propulsive movements close to the body centre line
6. Part practice Moderate	Kick, using a DRAG BELT, 200 metres on FRONT CRAWL	Work hard from the hips and keep the toes pointing mainly backwards

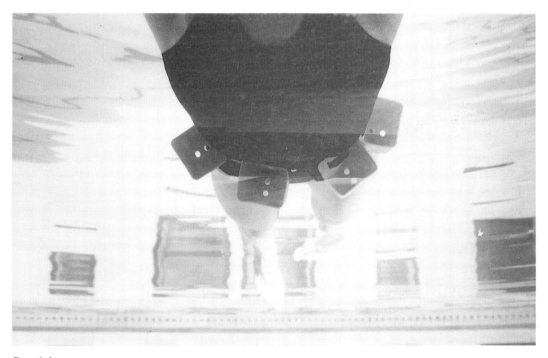

Drag belt.

Phase/Pace	Practice	Focus
7. Full stroke Moderate to fast	Swim 3 × 50 metres DESCENDING SET (SPEED) on FRONT CRAWL on 1 minute; swim the first 50 metres at a moderate pace, and swim faster with each succeeding 50 metres	Speed up the swims by speeding up the propulsive arm movements
8. Full stroke Moderate	Swim 4 × 25 metres INTERVAL on BUTTERFLY DOLPHIN on 40 seconds	Remember to drop the head as you swing the arms round and over the water surface
9. Cool-down, full stroke Slow	Swim 200 metres on FRONT CRAWL	Control the recovery and enter through the fingertips

QUESTIONS

1. Did you enter cleanly?
2. Did you find it easy to change speed?
3. Did you maintain a constant pace?
4. Did you swim faster on the second 25 metres?
5. Did you maintain a fast pace?
6. Did you maintain a constant pace?
7. Did you realise that phases 1 to 7 are pyramidal? (i.e. 150 metres to 300 metres and back to 150 metres)
8. Did you clear the water surface easily?
9. Did you enter cleanly even though you felt tired?

EXAMPLE 7

MAIN STROKE: Individual medley strokes.
SECOND STROKE: Own choice.
DISTANCE: 1900 metres.
OTHER SKILLS: Butterfly open turn.
EQUIPMENT: Float or kick board and pull buoy, clock or watch.

Phase/Pace	Practice	Focus
1. Warm-up, full stroke Slow	Swim 150 metres on BACK CRAWL	Recover the arms high and close to the ears
2. Full stroke Moderate	Swim 200 metres on INDIVIDUAL MEDLEY; swim 50 metres on each stroke	Breathe regularly every arm cycle
3. Turning	Water at shoulder level; swim on BUTTERFLY DOLPHIN to the pool side from a distance of 5 metres and practise a butterfly open turn, (practise for 5 minutes)	Touch the wall with both hands simultaneously and at the same level; turn, release the arms and sink on the side. Stretch away from the wall as you twist onto the front
4. Full stroke Moderate	Swim 3 × 50 metres INTERVAL on BUTTERFLY DOLPHIN on 80 seconds	Initiate the leg action from the hips and concentrate on kicking both upwards and downwards
5. Part practice Moderate	Kick 200 metres on INDIVIDUAL MEDLEY; swim 50 metres on each stroke	Keep the toes pointing mainly backwards on the crawl-type strokes and pointing mainly outwards on the breast stroke
6. Part practice Moderate	Pull 200 metres on INDIVIDUAL MEDLEY; swim 25 metres on each stroke and then repeat	Inhale at the same point every arm cycle
7. Full stroke and part practice Moderate	Swim, kick and pull 400 metres OVERDISTANCE on BREAST STROKE; swim 50 metres on breast stroke, kick 25 metres on breast stroke with the arms extended in front, pull 25 metres on breast stroke with a dolphin leg kick and then repeat	Accelerate all propulsive leg and arm movements
8. Full stroke All-out	Swim 4 × 25 metres SPRINT on BREAST STROKE (rest for 1 minute between each 25 metres)	Kick with the arms almost extended in front and start to pull before the legs have come together

Phase/Pace	Practice	Focus
9. Full stroke Moderate	Swim 4 × 75 metres INTERVAL with BI-LATERAL BREATHING on FRONT CRAWL (rest for 25 seconds between each 75 metres)	Concentrate on turning the head smoothly to the side that is not the usual breathing side
10. Cool-down, full stroke Slow	Swim 200 metres OWN CHOICE STROKE	Maintain slow but controlled limb movements

QUESTIONS

1. Did you loosen up your shoulder joints?
2. Did you get into a breathing rhythm on all strokes?
3. Did you touch and turn quickly?
4. Did you get the legs working?
5. Did you control the position of the feet?
6. Did you maintain the breathing rhythm?
7. Did you maintain a moderate pace on each aspect of the swim?
8. Did you recover enough to sprint each 25 metres?
9. Did you breathe every third arm stroke all the way?
10. Did you cool-down on the selected stroke?

EXAMPLE 8

MAIN STROKE: Back crawl.
SECOND STROKES: Own choice.
DISTANCE: 1900 metres.
OTHER SKILLS: None.
EQUIPMENT: Fins, clock or watch.

Phase/Pace	Practice	Focus
1. Warm-up, full stroke Slow	Swim 150 metres OWN CHOICE	Concentrate on working the joints
2. Full stroke and part practice Moderate	Swim, pull and kick 400 metres OVERDISTANCE on BACK CRAWL; swim 100 metres on back crawl, kick 100 metres on back crawl with the arms extended beyond the head, pull 100 metres on back crawl with occasional leg kicks and alternate each 25 metres the legs and the left arm and the legs and the right arm for the last 100 metres on back crawl	Even though the face is clear of the water all the time, it is important to breathe on a regular basis
3. Full stroke Moderate – fast	Swim 8 × 50 metres INTERVAL on BACK CRAWL on 1 minute 5 seconds, or 1 minute 10 seconds	Pull and push the hands along the body in an up and down movement; by rolling gently towards the propulsive arm the hand stays beneath the water surface
4. Full stroke Slow	Swim 100 metres OWN CHOICE STROKE	Establish a slow stroke rhythm breathing every arm cycle
5. Full stroke Fast	Start and swim 4 × 50 metres INTERVAL on BACK CRAWL on 1 minute or 1 minute 5 seconds (select a time 5 seconds faster than in phase 3)	Hug the side of the pool in a tight tuck position and explode backwards and upwards; swing the arms round to a position beyond the head and enter through the fingertips with the body slightly arched
6. Full stroke Slow	Swim 100 metres OWN CHOICE	Maintain a slow stroke rhythm and a regular breathing cycle
7. Full stroke All-out	Swim 4 × 25 metres BROKEN-SWIM (5 seconds rest between each 25 metres)	Recover the straight arms in a fast controlled movement

Phase/Pace	Practice	Focus
8. Part practice\
\
Moderate	Kick, using FINS, 250 metres on a CRAWL TYPE KICK (i.e. back crawl, front crawl, butterfly dolphin)	Work hard from the hips and kick more slowly than usual
9. Cool-down, full stroke\
\
Slow	Swim 200 metres OWN CHOICE STROKE	Work all limb movements slowly but steadily

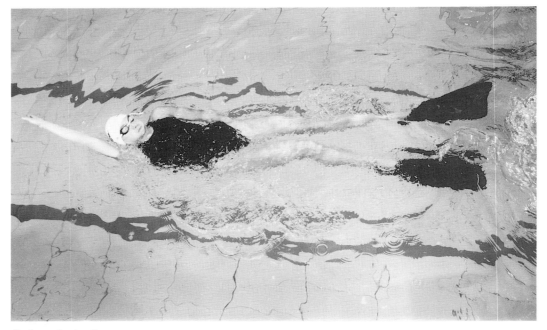

Back crawl using fins.

QUESTIONS

1. Did you warm-up?
2. Did you adjust quickly to the part practices?
3. Are you developing an 'S' movement?
4. Did you recover?
5. Did you manage the faster time?
6. Did you recover?
7. Did you swim 'all-out'?
8. THERE IS ALWAYS A DANGER OF FINS FLICKING SWIMMERS IN THE EYES SO IT IS IMPORTANT THAT 'FIN SWIMMING' IS CARRIED OUT IN A LANE SEPARATE FROM OTHER SWIMMERS
9. Did you take it easy?

EXAMPLE 9

MAIN STROKE: Front crawl.
SECOND STROKES: Own choice.
DISTANCE: 2000 metres.
OTHER SKILLS: None.
EQUIPMENT: Training tube, hand paddles, drag belt, drag suit, float or kick board and pull buoy,
clock or watch.

Phase/Pace	Practice	Focus
1. Warm-up, full stroke Slow	Swim 150 metres OWN CHOICE STROKE	Loosen up the joints
2. Full stroke Moderate and fast	Swim 300 metres FARTLEK on FRONT CRAWL; alternate moderate and fast swims, changing the speed after each 50 metres	Sharpen up the propulsive and recovery movements for the fast 50 metres
3. Full stroke Moderate	Swim, using a TRAINING TUBE, 250 metres on FRONT CRAWL	Concentrate on continuous arm actions
4. Part practice Moderate	Pull, using HAND PADDLES, 200 metres on FRONT CRAWL	Keep the elbows higher than the hands during the propulsive movements
5. Kick Moderate	Kick, using a DRAG BELT, 150 metres on FRONT CRAWL	Work hard on the upward movements and keep the leg actions shallow
6. Full stroke Fast	Swim 100 metres on FRONT CRAWL	Move the hands backwards in a curved path close to the centre line of the body.
7. Full stroke Fast	Swim 3 × 50 metres INTERVAL on 55 seconds	Pull and push vigorously and recover the arms in a fast, controlled movement
8. Full stroke Fast	Swim 8 × 25 metres INTERVAL on 25 seconds *or* 30 seconds	Maintain a fast stroke rhythm
9. Full stroke Moderate	Swim, using a DRAG SUIT, 250 metres on FRONT CRAWL	Maintain a regular leg kick with steady, continuous arm actions
10. Cool-down, full stroke Slow	Swim 250 metres on any 2 STROKES; organise in any way as long as you swim 125 metres on each stroke	Perform the stroke at a speed that just maintains the near horizontal body position

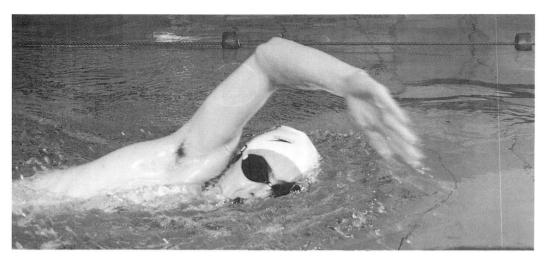

Front crawl recovery showing high elbow position.

QUESTIONS

1. Do you feel prepared for the next phase?
2. Did you maintain the fast pace?
3. Did you keep a steady arm rhythm going?
4. Did you keep the elbows up?
5. Did you keep the legs close to the water surface?
6. Did you maintain a fast controlled pace?
7. Did you manage this phase?
8. Did you get some rest at the end of each 25 metres?
9. What difference did you notice?
10. Did you swim in an easy and relaxed way?

EXAMPLE 10

MAIN STROKES: Own choice.
SECOND STROKES: Butterfly dolphin, own choice.
DISTANCE: 2000 metres.
OTHER SKILLS: None.
EQUIPMENT: Wrist weights, drag ring, float or kick board and pull buoy, clock or watch.

Phase/Pace	Practice	Focus
1. Warm-up, full stroke Slow	Swim 150 metres on 6 OWN CHOICE STROKES; 25 metres on each stroke	Breathe every arm cycle whatever the stroke
2. Full stroke Moderate	Swim 200 metres, using a DRAG RING, on MAIN STROKE	Accelerate the hands throughout the propulsive movements
3. Full stroke Moderate	Swim 250 metres on SECOND MAIN STROKE	Feel for a 'hold' on the water as the hands accelerate
4. Full stroke Moderate	Swim 300 metres on THIRD MAIN STROKE	Propulsive movements are vigorous
5. Part practice Moderate	Pull, using WRIST WEIGHTS, 350 metres on MAIN STROKE	Control all hand and wrist actions
6. Part practice Moderate	Kick 400 metres on your 3 MAIN STROKES; organise in any way as long as you swim a minimum of 100 metres on each stroke	Kick close to the water surface on the crawl-type strokes and streamline the legs at the end of the breast stroke propulsive movement
7. Full stroke Fast	Swim 3 × 50 metres on BUTTERFLY DOLPHIN on 1 minute 10 seconds or 1 minute 20 seconds	Concentrate on a continuous arm action with no pause when the arms are extended in front of the body
8. Cool-down, full stroke Slow	Swim 200 metres on MAIN STROKE	Slow down all limb movements

QUESTIONS

1. Can you swim 6 strokes?
2. Did you feel the pressure on the hands?
3. Did you 'hold' the water?
4. Did you feel the power in the hands?
5. Did you have to work hard?

6. Did you do the 400 metres continuously?
7. Did you maintain a fast pace on the last 50 metres?
8. Did you still maintain a stroke rhythm?

SOMETHING DIFFERENT

EXAMPLE 11

MAIN STROKES: Front crawl, breast stroke.
TIMED ACTIVITY: 10 minutes.
DISTANCE: 1225 metres.
OTHER SKILLS: Treading water, sculling, ball passing, plunge dive, surface dive, towing.

Phase/Pace	Practice	Focus
1. Find a partner		
2. Warm-up, full stroke Slow	Swim 150 metres on FRONT CRAWL with your partner	Look in a forwards and downwards direction in the non-breathing stage of the arm action
3. Full stroke Moderate	Swim 200 metres on BREAST STROKE, TREAD WATER (5 minutes), SCULL 10 metres HEAD OR FEET FIRST and swim 200 metres on FRONT CRAWL; this is a continuous sequence and to be performed without touching the bottom or the side of the pool	Swim clockwise or anti-clockwise in the lane and tread water and scull in the deep water
4. Ball skills (partner)	Deep water: pick up a ball and pass to your partner (5 minutes)	Pick up the ball by sliding the palm of the flat hand under the ball; hold the ball above the shoulder with a bent arm and straighten the arm to pass
5. Dive, swim and surface dive Moderate	Deep water: plunge dive, swim 50 metres OWN CHOICE STROKE (surface diving and swimming two or three metres underwater on two occasions), tow your partner 25 metres	Tense and streamline the body and limbs for the flight, entry and glide of the plunge dive; swim, pike vigorously and then lift the legs in line with the trunk to surface dive; swim underwater using an adapted breast stroke or dog's paddle that includes a push to the hips in the propulsive arm movements
6. Full stroke (partner) Moderate	Swim 400 metres on FRONT CRAWL and BREAST STROKE; swim *either* next to *or* behind your partner for the first 200 metres on FRONT CRAWL and swim *either* next to or in front of your partner for the second 200 metres on BREAST STROKE	Use your partner as the pacemaker for the first 200 metres and be the pacemaker for the second 200 metres

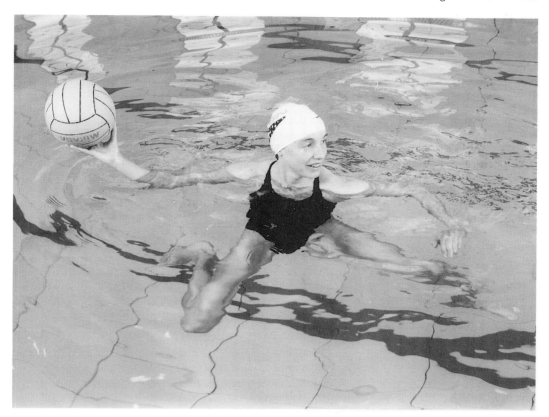

Ball skill using an egg-beater kick.

Phase/Pace	Practice	Focus
7. Cool-down, full stroke Slow	Swim 200 metres on OWN CHOICE STROKE	Swim slowly at your own pace

QUESTIONS

1. Is your partner about your standard?
2. Did you follow or lead your partner?
3. Did you plan the sequence?
4. Did you keep it going without hanging on to the ball or the pool side?
5. Did your partner try the sequence?
6. Did you keep together?
7. Which is your most comfortable stroke?

SOME SIMPLY ORGANISED LEVEL IV WORKOUTS

1. Swim 200 metres, warm-up,   SLOW
   Swim 800 metres
   OVERDISTANCE,   MODERATE
   Pull 400 metres
   OVERDISTANCE,   MODERATE
   Kick 400 metres
   OVERDISTANCE,   MODERATE
   Swim 200 metres, cool-down,   SLOW
   Total 2000 metres

2. Swim 200 metres, warm-up,   SLOW
   Swim 2 × 200 metres, on 4
   minutes,   MODERATE
   Pull 4 × 100 metres on 2
   minutes,   MODERATE
   Kick 400 metres,   MODERATE
   Swim 200 metres Individual
   Medley,   MODERATE
   (50 metres on each stroke)
   Swim 8 × 25 metres on 30
   seconds,   MODERATE
   Swim 200 metres, cool-down,   SLOW
   Total 2000 metres

3. Swim 200 metres, warm-up,   SLOW
   Swim 4 × 100 metres, 40 seconds
   rest,   MODERATE
   Swim 8 × 50 metres, 25 seconds
   rest,   MODERATE
   Swim 10 × 25 metres, 10 seconds
   rest,   MODERATE
   Pull 200 metres,   MODERATE
   Kick 150 metres,   MODERATE
   Swim 200 metres, cool-down,   SLOW
   Total 1800 metres

4. Swim 150 metres, warm-up,   SLOW
   Swim 1500 metres
   OVERDISTANCE,   MODERATE
   Swim 150 metres,   SLOW
   Total 1800 metres

SELECT YOUR OWN STROKES AND TRY TO
COMPLETE WITHIN 60 MINUTES.

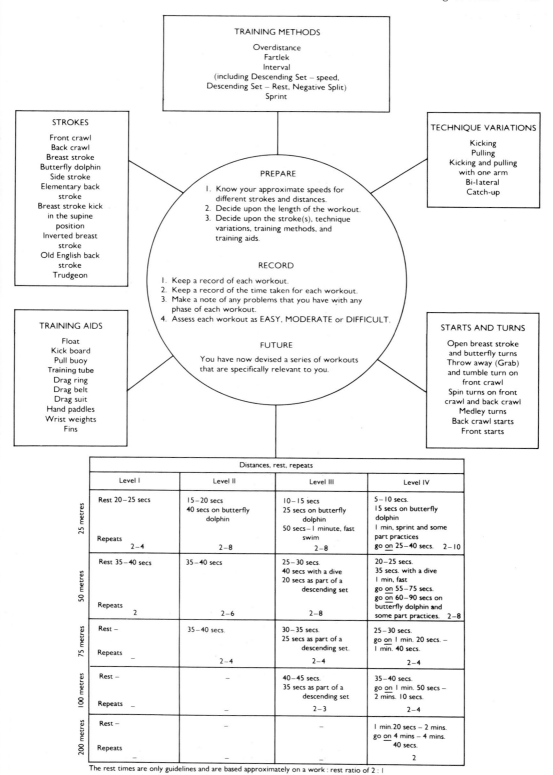

TRAINING METHODS

Overdistance
Fartlek
Interval
(including Descending Set – speed,
Descending Set – Rest, Negative Split)
Sprint

STROKES

Front crawl
Back crawl
Breast stroke
Butterfly dolphin
Side stroke
Elementary back
stroke
Breast stroke kick
in the supine
position
Inverted breast
stroke
Old English back
stroke
Trudgeon

TECHNIQUE VARIATIONS

Kicking
Pulling
Kicking and pulling
with one arm
Bi-lateral
Catch-up

PREPARE

1. Know your approximate speeds for
   different strokes and distances.
2. Decide upon the length of the workout.
3. Decide upon the stroke(s), technique
   variations, training methods, and
   training aids.

RECORD

1. Keep a record of each workout.
2. Keep a record of the time taken for each workout.
3. Make a note of any problems that you have with any
   phase of each workout.
4. Assess each workout as EASY, MODERATE or DIFFICULT.

FUTURE

You have now devised a series of workouts
that are specifically relevant to you.

TRAINING AIDS

Float
Kick board
Pull buoy
Training tube
Drag ring
Drag belt
Drag suit
Hand paddles
Wrist weights
Fins

STARTS AND TURNS

Open breast stroke
and butterfly turns
Throw away (Grab)
and tumble turn on
front crawl
Spin turns on front
crawl and back crawl
Medley turns
Back crawl starts
Front starts

Distances, rest, repeats			
Level I	Level II	Level III	Level IV
25 metres Rest 20–25 secs Repeats 2–4	15–20 secs 40 secs on butterfly dolphin 2–8	10–15 secs 25 secs on butterfly dolphin 50 secs–1 minute, fast swim 2–8	5–10 secs. 15 secs on butterfly dolphin 1 min, sprint and some part practices go on 25–40 secs. 2–10
50 metres Rest 35–40 secs Repeats 2	35–40 secs 2–6	25–30 secs. 40 secs with a dive 20 secs as part of a descending set 2–8	20–25 secs. 35 secs. with a dive 1 min, fast go on 55–75 secs. go on 60–90 secs on butterfly dolphin and some part practices. 2–8
75 metres Rest – Repeats –	35–40 secs. 2–4	30–35 secs. 25 secs as part of a descending set. 2–4	25–30 secs. go on 1 min. 20 secs. – 1 min. 40 secs. 2–4
100 metres Rest – Repeats –	– –	40–45 secs. 35 secs as part of a descending set 2–3	35–40 secs. go on 1 min. 50 secs – 2 mins. 10 secs. 2–4
200 metres Rest – Repeats –	– –	– –	1 min.20 secs – 2 mins. go on 4 mins – 4 mins. 40 secs. 2

The rest times are only guidelines and are based approximately on a work : rest ratio of 2 : 1

*Figure 21 Construct you own
workout.*

APPENDIX A

EXAMPLE OF A LEVEL III WORKOUT (SEE PAGE 78, EXAMPLE 10) PRESENTED IN ABBREVIATED FORM

Phase/Pace		Practice	Focus
1. Swim	S	200 { 100 SS / 50 EB / 50BrS	Timing
2. Turning		5 mins – BC	Legs out and over
3. Pull	M	300 – BC	Accelerate propulsive movement
4. Kick	M	200 – BC	Knees under
5. Swim	M	300 – BC	'S' movement.
6. Swim / Tread water / Swim	S	250 – FC / – 3 mins. / 250 – BC	Head position

QUESTIONS

1. Are you improving the strokes?
2. Did you get the legs out of the water?
3. Did you feel the water pressure on the hands?
4. Did you keep the knees under?
5. Did you 'hold' the water with the hands?
6. Were you in control of the various head positions?

Key: SS = Side stroke.
EB = Elementary back stroke.
Br S = Breast stroke kick in the supine position.
BC = Back crawl.
S = Slow.
M = Moderate.

Other examples of abbreviated forms

FC = Front crawl.
Br = Breast stroke.
Bu D = Butterfly dolphin.
Bu B = Butterfly breast stroke.
OEB = Old English back stroke.
IB = Inverted breast stroke.
IM = Individual medley.
F = Fast.
Alt = Alternating.
OvD = Overdistance.

FTK = Fartlek.
IT = Interval training.
DeS (r) = Descending set (rest).
DeS (s) = Descending set (speed).
Ne.S = Negative split.
Br-Sw = Broken-swim.
Sp = Sprint.
Bi-L = Bi-lateral.
Ca-up = Catch-up.

4 × 100 IT on 2 mins = 4 repetitions of 100 metres going every 2 minutes.

4 × 75 IT R 25 secs = 4 repetitions of 75 metres resting for 25 seconds between each repetition.

4 × 50 DeS (r) 30, 25, 20 = 4 repetitions of 50 metres resting for 30 seconds after the first 50 metres, 25 seconds after the second 50 metres and 20 seconds after the third 50 metres.

4 × 50 DeS (s) = 4 repetitions of 50 metres swimming each 50 metres faster than the previous one.

4 × 50 NeS on 65 = 4 repetitions of 50 metres swimming the second 25 metres of each 50 metres faster than the first 25 metres and still going every 65 seconds.

4 × 25 Br-Sw R 5 secs = 4 repetitions of 25 metres resting for 5 seconds between each 25 metres.

400 FTK, Alt.S a F ea 25 = Swim 400 metres Fartlek alternating a slow and fast length every 25 metres.

APPENDIX B

PHYSIOLOGICAL RESPONSES TO SWIMMING TRAINING

K. Sharman
Loughborough University of Technology

A study was carried out at Loughborough University to investigate the effects of 6 weeks' training on the fitness of recreational swimmers. Twenty six non-competitive, untrained swimmers (18 females and 8 males, aged 19–26) acted as subjects for the study. The swimmers were divided into two matched groups, experimental and control. The experimental group trained for 40 minutes three times a week, giving a total of 12 hours of swimming training. The training undertaken was a progressive programme comprising sessions of mixed strokes and varying work intensity. The schedules used were based on those presented in this book. In the initial training sessions the experimental group covered approximately 900 yards in the 40 minutes (schedules taken from Level II of the programme); by the end of the six weeks they were completing Level IV sessions of 1400 yards. No stroke tuition was given to the

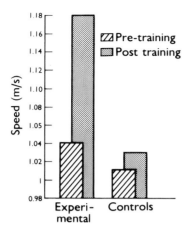

Figure A1 Changes in maximal performance before and after training in experimental group and in control group.

group as there was no intention of changing skill levels. The control group continued their usual swimming activity of low-intensity, distance type training.

Physiological measures, a 100 yard maximum effort time trial and submaximal tests were performed before and after the period of training. The 100 yard swim time was also expressed as an average swim speed (Vmax, m/s). The submaximal test consisted of swimming at 60, 70, 80 and 90% of the initial 100 yard speed; thus the same speeds were swum before and after the training programme. Any physiological changes in response to the submaximal swimming test could then be assessed. A small blood sample (25 μl and duplicate) was then taken after each submaximal swim and analysed for blood lactic concentrations. A decrease in the concentration of blood lactic acid produced when swimming at the same speed after training was taken to be indicative of an improvement in the endurance fitness of the individual.

After the 6 week training period both groups improved their 100 yard swimming time and consequently their Vmax, as shown in Table A1 and Fig. A1. The experimental group improved their mean swim speed from 1.04 ± 0.03 to 1.16 ± 0.05 m/s[1]; this was a significantly greater margin than that achieved by the control group ($p<0.01$). Blood lactic acid concentrations were decreased significantly at the set submaximal speeds for both groups after the 6 weeks of swimming training (Table A2 and Fig. A2). This fall in blood lactic acid concentration was significantly larger at the 90% swimming speed for the experimental group ($p<0.05$), as shown in Fig. A3.

The improved 100 yard time and decreased submaximal lactate values shown by the experimental group were attributed to an improvement in swimming fitness. This change, in turn, may be attributed to participation in a regular, mixed intensity, progressive swimming training programme. The results of the study therefore show that an improvement in swimming fitness, traditionally assessed by improvements in maximum performance tests, can also be reflected by submaximal tests. These tests comprise the analysis of blood lactic acid concentrations at set submaximal swimming speeds before and after training.

TABLE A1

Summary of mean swimming performance test changes for all subjects

	Experiment	Control
Pre-training		
Maximum 100 yard time (s)	88.48 ± 2.91	91.29 ± 3.83
Maximum 100 yard speed (m/s)	1.04 ± 0.03	1.01 ± 0.04
Post-training		
Maximum 100 yard time (s)	79.84 ± 3.11	89.36 ± 3.70
Maximum 100 yard speed (m/s)	1.16 ± 0.05	1.03 ± 0.04
Change %	+10.04*	+2.51

* $p < 0.01$

TABLE A2

Mean lactic acid concentrations (mMol/l) at a range of submaximal swimming speeds before and after training

	Percentage of pre-training Vmax			
	60	**70**	**80**	**90**
Experiment				
Before training	1.20 ± 0.97	1.90 ± 0.86	2.57 ± 1.38	4.06 ± 2.10
After training	1.10 ± 0.54	1.42 ± 0.76	1.74 ± 0.82	2.53 ± 1.10
Change in value	0.079 ± 0.74	0.44 ± 0.71	0.87 ± 1.25	1.52 ± 1.47
Percentage decrease	8.3	25.3	32.3	37.7
Control				
Before training	1.46 ± 0.71	2.25 ± 1.13	3.01 ± 1.59	4.51 ± 1.96
After training	1.08 ± 0.56	1.90 ± 0.92	2.34 ± 1.25	3.84 ± 2.04
Change in value	0.39 ± 0.41	0.38 ± 0.55	0.57 ± 0.86	0.72 ± 0.57
Percentage decrease	26.0	15.6	22.3	14.9

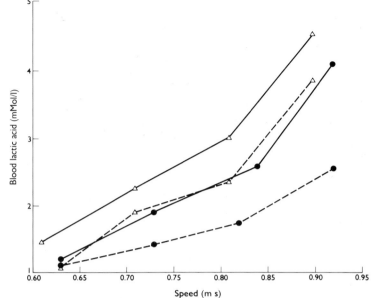

Figure A2 Blood lactic acid concentrations before and after training in all subjects. ●———● = Experimental group before training; ●– – –● = Experimental group after training; △———△ = Control group before training; △_ _ _△ = Control group after training.

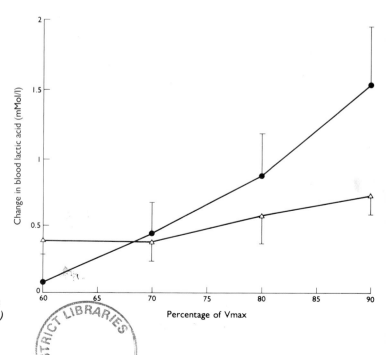

Figure A3 Change in blood lactic acid concentrations after training in experimental (●) and in control (△) groups.